How to Stop Overthinking Now

Easy Techniques to Calm Your Mind, Stop Negative Thoughts, and (Finally) Relieve Stress With Positive Psychology Secrets

Logan Mind

A Gift for You!

Emotional Intelligence for Social Success

Here's what you'll find in the **book**:

• Techniques to enhance your **social skills**

• Strategies to master your **emotions**

• Tips for improving your **interactions** and relationships

Just click or follow the link below to start your **journey** towards social success:

https://pxl.to/loganmindfreebook

Pick up your 3 FREE EXTRAS too!

These extras are designed to supplement your reading **experience** and help you get the most out of the book. They provide practical **tools** that you can use to apply the concepts discussed in the book to your daily life.

The extras are:

- A downloadable and practical PDF 21-Day **Challenge** for the book

- 101+ Affirmations for Peaceful Minds

- Instant Calm Mind Checklist

Just click or follow the link below to gain instant **access** to the extras:

https://pxl.to/8-htson-lm-extras

Help Me!

When you support an independent author, you're supporting a **dream**.

When you're done reading and if you're satisfied, please consider leaving an honest **review**. Your **feedback** not only helps other readers discover the book but also aids in my growth as a writer.

If you've got suggestions for improvements, I'd be delighted to hear from you. Just shoot an email to the contacts you can find at the link below.

Alternatively, you can scan the QR code provided to easily access the review page.

Your review matters.

It only takes a few seconds, but your **voice** has a huge **impact**, encouraging and inspiring storytellers like myself to continue sharing our worlds and words with you.

Thanks for being a part of this **journey**.

Visit this link to leave feedback:

https://pxl.to/8-htson-lm-review

Join my Review Team!

Thank you for taking the time to read my **book**. Your support means the world to me. I'm excited to invite you to join my ARC (Advanced Reader Copy) **team**. As a member, you'll receive free copies of my upcoming **books** before they hit the shelves. Your honest **feedback** will be invaluable and help shape my work for future readers.

Becoming part of the **team** is an easy process:

• Click on "Join Review Team"

• Sign Up to BookSprout

• Get notified every time I release a new book

Check out the team at this link:

https://pxl.to/loganmindteam

Introduction

Have you ever found yourself lying awake at night, unable to **turn off** your thoughts? Maybe you've replayed a conversation over and over, wondering if you said the right thing. If that sounds like you, this book is like your **guide** to help you break free from that frustrating cycle of overthinking.

Overthinking doesn't just keep you up at night. It seeps into your daily life, making you second-guess yourself, worry about things that won't happen, and even cause stress and anxiety. It's a habit, almost like an uninvited guest, that makes everything feel more complicated than it needs to be.

I wrote this book to show you that there are ways to take **control** of your thoughts and finally find some peace of mind. We're going to talk about a bunch of strategies and little tricks that are based on Positive Psychology. I wanted to create something practical, something you can actually use right away to start feeling better.

But first, let's chat a bit about this whole overthinking thing. It's not just random thoughts running wild in your brain; there's actually some **psychology** behind it. Maybe you're triggered by stress, or perhaps it's tied to anxiety. Maybe you've just got into the habit of worrying too much. You'll get a better understanding of why you overthink and how it's affecting your mental health. It's kind of interesting when you see why your brain does what it does.

I've spent years studying human behavior and showing people how to communicate better and live healthier lives. I've worked with high-powered execs, guided them, seen firsthand how these tactics make a real difference. It's all about blending practical advice with real, proven techniques. And trust me, if they can make a difference for busy professionals, they can definitely work for you.

One of the biggest hurdles with overthinking is that it forms a stubborn cycle that's tough to break. It's like being caught in a loop of stress and anxiety. But we'll work through ways to recognize these patterns, understand where they're coming from, and learn how to dismantle them step by step. Once you see how it all works, it becomes a bit easier to manage.

And yes, I get it – you've probably tried a lot of things. Maybe you've read similar stuff, followed advice that just didn't stick. Perhaps you think you're just too wired this way and there's no way out. But I want to show you that with a few intentional shifts and practical exercises, breaking free from overthinking really is possible. I've seen people turn things around with just these concepts.

The **strategies** we'll go through aren't to make you feel overwhelmed by even more "things to do" or hoops to jump through. They're straightforward, meant to fit into your day without adding extra stress. From grounding exercises to thought diffusion strategies, these are everyday tools that make managing your mind simpler. You'll find ways to stop negative thoughts right in their tracks and bring a bit more calm into your life.

Think about it – being able to wake up, go through your day without those constant nagging thoughts holding you back. It's about getting through your tasks without the endless mental dialogue slowing you down.

People often argue that overthinking is an ingrained part of who they are, that it's just personality or some deeply-rooted trait that can't be changed. But that's not true. **Mindsets** can shift, and you can start thinking differently if you just look at things with fresh eyes and approach your patterns of thought with new strategies.

So why did I write this book? Because I believe everyone deserves that clarity and peace. It's not about never having a stressful thought again, but about finding ways to manage them better. Who wouldn't want the tools to handle their thoughts more effectively and reduce unnecessary stress?

In our time together, we'll cover an array of helpful methods tailored to help calm your mind. This is more than just advice. It's a practical **guide**, meant to be picked apart and pieced together to fit your life.

At the end of the day, this book is a way to give you peace of mind and bring a bit more tranquility to your everyday routine. By integrating Positive Psychology principles, these strategies offer you alleviation from the burdens your thoughts may have on you.

Ready to step into a more relaxed, thought-controlled day-to-day life? By diving into these chapters, you're taking the first step toward calming your mind and letting go of those looping thoughts.

Let's get **started**!

Chapter 1: Understanding Overthinking

Ever find yourself **thinking** way too much about something? Like, over and over until it's all you can focus on? I used to do that a lot. In this chapter, we're gonna chat about what overthinking really is and why your **brain** goes into overdrive sometimes. There's a lot behind it, stuff you might not even realize. You'll get hooked on knowing the **psychology** that fuels it—makes you go, "Whoa, so that's why it happens."

I'll also share some common things that **trigger** overthinking—stuff that's probably right under your nose. And, yeah, we'll see what it does to your **mental** health—spoiler, it ain't too pretty. But stick around, 'cause understanding this stuff is like finding out a hidden **superpower**. Trust me, you'll want to read more and figure out how to turn the tables on overthinking. Ready to get **started**?

You're about to dive into the nitty-gritty of overthinking. It's not just about worrying too much; it's a whole **process** that can take over your mind. We'll explore why your brain sometimes feels like it's stuck on repeat, playing the same thoughts over and over again. You'll get the inside scoop on what's happening up there in your noggin when overthinking kicks in.

Think of this chapter as your personal guide to understanding why you sometimes can't shut off those pesky thoughts. We'll break it down in a way that'll make you go, "Oh, that makes sense!" By the time you're done, you'll have a better grip on what's going on in your head and why. It's like getting a backstage pass to your own mind.

So, buckle up and get ready to learn about the ins and outs of overthinking. It might just change the way you look at your thoughts forever. Let's jump in and start unraveling this mental mystery together!

What is Overthinking?

Ever found yourself going over the same thoughts again and again, like a broken record? That's what we'll talk about first: **overthinking**. When you obsessively replay thoughts in your head that don't really lead anywhere, that's overthinking. It might start with something small, like a worry about a meeting or a comment someone made. Before you know it, you're **spiraling**— imagining worst-case scenarios, second-guessing yourself, and getting more anxious. And what's the kicker? None of that mental gymnastics helps you make any decisions.

So why do you do this? Well, it can be your brain's way of trying to gain control or solve problems. But instead of solving things, it just makes you feel stuck. You're mentally **exhausted**, and you haven't actually moved forward.

Now, let's talk about the difference between thinking stuff through in a healthy way and getting stuck in harmful thoughts. Picture yourself planning a trip. You consider where to go, what to pack, ideal travel dates... useful stuff. But if you're overthinking? You'll worry about flight delays, lost luggage, hotel horror stories. You'll go in circles until planning feels like torture. Knowing the line separating the two— that's important.

Healthy thinking is like a road trip with a map. You have a **destination** and take steps to get there. Overthinking is driving in circles, feeling lost, not knowing which way to turn. One helps you make sound decisions, the other leaves you frazzled and uncertain. Being stuck in neutral isn't helping anybody.

Now, about these sneaky mental processes that mess with your head. When you overthink, your mind leans on certain mental habits that sneakily make things worse. **Catastrophizing** is one— thinking something tiny will snowball into a monstrous problem. Like, a friend doesn't text back and you think, "They hate me!"

There's also this thing called **analysis paralysis**, where you're so caught up in weighing every possible outcome that you do... nothing. Maybe you've got an important decision to make, like getting a new job or moving to a new city, but instead, you're stuck— constantly rehashing details without taking any action. Instead of simplifying and seeing basic steps, you're buried beneath endless "what ifs."

And don't forget about seeking **reassurance**. You might feel the need to ask ten friends what they would do in your situation, but this can keep you from learning to trust your own judgment. You end up relying more on everyone's opinions than what feels right to you. It's like adding layers to the mess— more opinions, more confusion, less clarity.

Overthinking is a messy maze, and it does a real number on your mental health. It sucks away joy, tweaks you into being overly cautious, anxious— even panicky. Once you start to notice these unhelpful habits, though, you can begin to steer your brain in a healthier direction. Switch lanes from overthinking to plain-old thinking, and you'll find driving through life's decisions a whole lot smoother.

So, in a nutshell, overthinking traps you in a cycle of worries that accomplish next to nothing and make you feel all sorts of bad. Healthy thinking helps you move forward with decisions. And recognizing the tricks your mind uses can set you on the path to better **mental health**. We've just dipped our toes into the topic of overthinking. It's like you're switching gears from obsessive loops to mindful decisions, bringing you one step closer to calm and clarity.

The Psychology Behind Overthinking

Let's **chat** about mental shortcuts. Have you ever found yourself stuck in a loop of thoughts, over and over? That's partly because your **brain** likes shortcuts. It's a bit like taking the same familiar path home even when there might be a quicker route. Your brain does this to save energy and time, but it also makes it really easy to fall into the trap of **overthinking**. You get used to certain patterns, and before you know it, you're trudging down the same old paths, getting nowhere fast.

For instance, you might think, "If I don't do this perfectly, everything will fall apart." This black-and-white **thinking** doesn't give you room to mess up or even just be average. It's exhausting, right? Your brain creates these shortcuts based on past **experiences** and learned behaviors. And because they're so ingrained, they're tough to shake. They almost feel automatic.

There's more to it, of course, and it ties in with your past. Yup, all those experiences you've had play a big role in why you can't stop thinking sometimes. Stuff you've been through teaches your brain how to react. If you've had a tough time with failure or criticism, your mind learns to be on alert, always watching for potential threats. This constant vigilance makes overthinking kind of your default mode.

Remember that time you made a mistake as a kid and got scolded? Moments like that leave marks. They tell your brain, 'Hey, we need to never let that happen again.' So you end up overanalyzing every little thing to avoid similar outcomes.

And it's not just the bad times, either. Even high expectations set by yourself or others can kickstart overthinking. Picture your brain storing all these tiny details and constantly picking through them to find what might go wrong or how things could be better. It's like a computer running too many programs at once, overheating your thoughts.

So, why does your brain keep running the same thoughts in a loop? Well, our brains are wired for repetition. They love patterns and routine. When you come across a **problem** or something that stresses you out, your brain rewinds the issue, playing it over and over, trying to find a solution. But here's the catch: sometimes there is no perfect solution, so you end up spinning your wheels, getting stuck in the same thoughts again and again.

Think of it like getting a song stuck in your head. Your brain picks it up and doesn't want to let go. Little triggers—like a word or a feeling—can start the tune playing, or in this case, start your worries running. Plus, the **emotional** charge tied to these thoughts gives them extra power. So, if it's something that makes you anxious, your mind just keeps churning on it, convinced it's too important to let go.

The parts of your brain involved here include the prefrontal cortex, your thinking cap if you will. It tries to plan and solve, but sometimes it overdoes it. And there's the amygdala, which handles emotions like fear and anxiety. When they team up, they turn you into an overthinking machine.

So, in essence, overthinking is a mix of mental shortcuts, your past baggage, and the brain's love for repetition. Once you understand this, you start seeing how they all feed each other. Recognizing this is the first step toward untangling those repetitive, **stress**-inducing thoughts.

Common Triggers for Overthinking

Let's talk about what usually kicks off those endless loops of thoughts. There's plenty of outside stuff that can set off **overthinking** episodes. Things like work, relationships, social media... you name it. Ever been at work with a mountain of tasks piling up? Yeah, that can do it. Or maybe it's a silly comment from a friend that you just can't shake off. It sticks in your **brain**, and you start replaying every possible angle of what they meant. Even scrolling through social media and seeing everyone's highlight reel can get you thinking that your life isn't measuring up. And don't forget the news. With all that's going on in the world, it's easy to get sucked into a whirlwind of thoughts about things way beyond your control.

But let's shift gears here—moving from these outside things to what's happening inside. It's not just the external stuff but also your personal **worries** and self-doubt. You've got things you fret about. It's like, maybe you've got concerns about your performance at work, or how friends and family see you. Self-doubt can kick you while you're down, making you question every choice, word, and action. Are you good enough? Did you make the right decision? These questions spiral until you're tangled in a web of your own making. And sometimes, these worries don't have a basis in reality—they're just your mind playing tricks on you. You start second-guessing your **decisions**, thinking you'll mess up somehow, even when there's no real proof to back that up.

Alright, shifting from self-doubt now... let's hit on another trigger—**fear** of the unknown. Not knowing what's going to happen next can really get your mind racing. If the future feels like this big, scary question mark, it's natural to start imagining all sorts of scenarios. And man, can those thoughts multiply. You're stuck thinking about how little control you have over what might or might not happen. Will things go your way? What if they don't? What if something goes horribly wrong? It's that need to anticipate every possibility that fuels overthinking. You think that if you can plan for every outcome, you'll be ready... but all you get is more **confusion** and less clarity.

In summary, it's these external events, along with your personal worries and the fear of the unknown, that really set the stage for overthinking. Recognizing these **triggers** is the first step to calming your mind. When you're aware, you can start to tweak how you respond to these situations and slowly, but surely, find some **peace** in the chaos.

The Impact of Overthinking on Mental Health

Ever felt like your mind just won't shut off? That's overthinking for you. It's not just a pesky habit – it's closely tied to **anxiety** disorders. When you overthink, your brain goes into overdrive, never taking a breather. This constant worry and those looping thoughts are like throwing fuel on the anxiety fire. You end up feeling more anxious because you keep chewing on the same problem over and over. Instead of moving forward, you're stuck in mental quicksand.

Overthinking isn't just annoying; it's downright dangerous. It takes a huge toll on your **mental health**. When you're constantly fretting about things that might or might not happen, it's tough to feel calm or happy. This kind of mental strain can make you more prone to other mental health issues, like depression. It's like putting your mind through a pressure cooker – eventually, it'll crack under the strain.

But it's not just about anxiety. Overthinking messes with your **brain** – literally. Ever had one of those nights when your thoughts are racing and you just can't sleep? That's overthinking messing with your shut-eye. **Sleep** is super important for overall brain function;

it's when your brain recharges. If you're tossing and turning all night, your brain doesn't get the rest it needs. You wake up tired and foggy, and this bad sleep cycle can mess up your concentration, memory, and even your mood during the day.

Overthinking can also lead to serious sleep disorders. Chronic insomnia, anyone? It's a cruel cycle: you worry about things which keeps you awake, and then you worry about not getting enough sleep. This never-ending loop can really mess up your overall brain function. A tired brain is a slow brain. You'll find it hard to remember things, make decisions, or even just think straight. Over time, this can make you pretty irritable and worn out.

Now, let's shift gears a bit and talk about the long-term effects of overthinking on **emotional health**. When you always overthink, everything feels like a burden. It changes the way you react to things. You might start to see everything through a lens of worry and doubt. It's not healthy. When your mind is always in overdrive, you lose out on actually living your life. Your **emotions** end up in chaos. You could feel anxious, sad, or even just plain numb.

This constant stress affects how you handle **relationships** too. You're exhausted, irritable, and struggle to enjoy the little moments. Long-term overthinking can lead to burnout. Your mind and body give up on you. Emotional exhaustion sets in. It's like running a marathon every single day. You can't keep up forever. Eventually, it affects your sense of self-worth and can lead to more severe issues like chronic depression or anxiety disorders.

So to wrap it all up, overthinking is more than just a few sleepless nights. It's a habit that hijacks your mental health, screws up your sleep, and messes with your emotional well-being in the long run. Breaking free from overthinking is crucial for your **mental health**. No small task, but it's clear why it's worth the effort.

In Conclusion

This chapter has given you valuable **insights** into the complex world of overthinking, equipping you with **knowledge** on how to better understand and manage it. By exploring the various elements that contribute to overthinking, you can begin to see just how **pervasive** and impactful it can be on your everyday life.

In this chapter, you've learned about the **definition** of overthinking and how it can lead to anxiety and indecision. You've also discovered the important differences between healthy reflection and harmful overthinking. You've seen how cognitive biases and past experiences can contribute to overthinking, and you've explored the **triggers** that often spark it, like personal insecurities and uncertainty. Additionally, you've gained an understanding of the negative **impact** of overthinking on mental health, including its effects on sleep and overall cognitive function.

By applying the lessons learned here, you can start to **recognize** when you're overthinking and take steps to manage it. Use this knowledge to cultivate a healthier mindset and reduce the hold that overthinking has over your life. With practice and **awareness**, you can pave the way for a more peaceful and productive mind. Keep pushing forward, and you can overcome the habit of overthinking!

Chapter 2: The Overthinking Cycle

Ever feel like your **mind's** a hamster on a wheel, always running but getting nowhere? I sure have. In this chapter, you'll take that mental hamster and show it who's boss. You won't just skim the surface; you'll learn to spot your **patterns** and tackle the gnawing **anxiety** that feeds them.

Imagine understanding your overthinking **habits** so well that you can pause them—like hitting mute on a noisy TV. Here's the kicker: You'll see how **stress** throws fuel on the overthinking fire, turning a tiny spark into a full-blown blaze.

Sound familiar? Thought so. But, we'll keep it simple, slicing through the thicket of **thoughts**, making way for sanity to peek through. You'll begin to sense how these anxious storms brew and learn to calm those pesky winds.

Ready to take **control**? Dive in, and let's turn this wheel into something way more **manageable**.

Identifying Your Overthinking Patterns

Ever felt like you're **trapped** in your own head, your thoughts looping endlessly? Knowing when you're overthinking is half the battle. Being aware of yourself helps you catch the moment your thoughts start spiraling. It's like noticing a storm brewing—you know it's coming, and you can get ready for it instead of being caught off guard.

You might not even realize you're overthinking until you're knee-deep in it. But if you can spot it early, you can nip it in the bud. Think about it: How often do you find yourself mulling over the same worry, dissecting it from every angle, getting lost in a web of "what-ifs"? Being **mindful**, catching yourself in these situations, brings you a step closer to calmness.

Now that we've set the stage for why awareness matters, let's dive into the nuts and bolts of overthinking itself.

Common overthinking patterns are like old friends you wish would quit visiting. Most of us have a few signature moves when it comes to overthinking. For example, you might get stuck in a cycle of **worry**. Your brain gets hooked on a concern and won't let it go, playing the same scene over and over like a movie stuck on repeat.

Another common one: over-analyzing. This is when you dissect every detail of a situation, trying to make sense of it until your brain feels like mush. It's like turning up the resolution on an image until it's just a bunch of blurry dots.

Catastrophizing is a biggie too. Ever taken a small problem and envisioned it leading to the end of the world? Your mind jumps from "I missed a deadline" to "I'm going to lose my job and end up living in a cardboard box." It's a slippery slope that leads straight to anxiety town.

We know these things take a toll on your mental health, but guess what often triggers these episodes? That's right, **emotions**.

Your emotional triggers play a sneaky role in starting the overthinking process. Imagine you're feeling stressed about a project at work. Nothing major, but it's enough to set your brain on a run. Next thing you know, you're questioning every decision you've ever made.

Anxiety, anger, sadness—they all light the fuse. You hear a negative comment, or maybe you get into a heated argument with a friend. Bang! Your mind goes off like fireworks, dissecting every phrase and action. It's tough. Emotions make overthinking feel necessary, like you're solving life's problems by examining each part up close.

Recognizing these **triggers** helps you prepare. That stress you feel? It's a sign. The argument circling in your mind like a hawk? Another sign. The upset voice in your head? Yep, another clue.

Understanding why it's so important to be aware of when you're overthinking, recognizing your common thinking patterns, and knowing your emotional triggers—these are key steps to cool down that overthinking engine. Start small, notice a pattern today, catch an overthink tomorrow. One step at a time, you start turning the **tide**.

Breaking Down the Overthinking Process

Let's chat about how the overthinking cycle actually works. It's like a chain reaction that starts with one small **trigger** - maybe it's a comment from someone, or an upcoming event. At first, it's just a fleeting thought. But before you know it, you're deep into analyzing every single detail. It's almost like you're building a snowball that just gets bigger and bigger.

And then, bam! You're trapped. You start creating **scenarios** and thinking about every possible outcome. What if things don't go as planned? What if something bad happens? This is where the whole process begins to spiral. Instead of focusing on what you can control, you're caught up imagining all sorts of outcomes. You're rehearsing conversations in your head, picturing worst-case scenarios, and stressing about things that might never even happen.

Now, let's not ignore the mental **traps** we fall into because of overthinking. It's like your mind sets up these tricky snares that keep you stuck. There's black-and-white thinking, where everything is either all good or all bad. No middle ground. It's either a win or a colossal failure. And let's not forget about mind-reading. You convince yourself you know what others are thinking about you, and it's never nice stuff. Another big trap is catastrophizing. You expect the worst possible thing to happen, blowing everything out of proportion. These mental traps? They fuel the overthinking fire, making it even harder to snap out of it.

Hold up, let's talk about how all this connects to something incredibly sneaky—negative **self-talk**. So, you're already in this cycle thanks to a trigger and mental traps. Throw in some critical self-talk, and you've got a perfect storm. You start telling yourself you're not good enough. You mess up; you're a failure. The voice in your head becomes your biggest critic. You're hard on yourself for not being able to predict the future or for making mistakes. It's like you've got an internal bully constantly beating you down.

And not just that—it's repetitive. The same harsh words again and again. Maybe you tell yourself you're a bad friend for not texting back right away. Or perhaps you think you're doomed to fail because you made a small mistake at work. You probably would never speak to a friend the way you talk to yourself, right? But here you are, creating a toxic cycle that's hard to break. The more harshly you talk to yourself, the more **anxious** and stressed you get, keeping the overthinking machine well-oiled and running.

So, the **process** goes like this: A simple trigger starts the whole thing. Then you're caught in mental traps. That leads to negative self-talk and pumps up the anxiety. It's a vicious cycle. Pretty tough to escape, but knowing how it works is the first step toward breaking free. Recognizing these steps won't magically solve everything, but it's a start. You've got the **roadmap**—now you can work on shutting down that overthinking **engine** and find some peace.

The Role of Anxiety in Overthinking

Have you ever noticed how **anxiety** and **overthinking** seem to be best buddies, always hanging out and making things worse? It all starts with a tiny worry. Maybe it's something you need to do or something that happened. It's on your mind, and you just can't shake it.

Your thoughts start to **spiral** because that little worry snowballs into a massive heap of stress and what-ifs. You find yourself thinking, "What if I can't fix this?" or "Will I ever get out of this?" Sounds foolish, right? But hey, everyone does this. Your brain sees a minor thing and decides to turn it into a full-blown drama.

And just like that, you're stuck. The anxiety grows, feeding on the overthinking, which grows right back. It's a **vicious cycle**, a loop you can't break by sheer willpower. It doesn't help that the more anxious you feel, the more you overthink. And the more you overthink, the more anxious you get. It's like a terrible feedback loop where you become your own worst enemy.

Guess what happens next? Your **body** decides to join the party. We all know that when our minds go haywire, our bodies can't just sit out. You start to shake, sweat, and feel your heart pounding in your chest like it's trying to escape. Sound familiar? That's your body reacting to your anxiety-driven overthinking. It's like having an argument between your brain and body that neither can win.

Think about it. You're so wrapped up in your thoughts, churning over them endlessly, it's no wonder your body gives the "code red."

Tight muscles, upset stomach, bad sleep - all invitations from anxiety. There's this domino effect: mind freaks out, body reacts, mind flees into more overthinking.

Anxiety also tricks you into thinking that more thinking will fix your problems. You feel like you've got to rethink everything, plan better, and prep for the worst. But nah! This just adds fuel to the fire. Your mind's buzzing like a swarm of bees - endless noise, not getting any gentler at all.

By this point, your body is tired... Physically tired, mentally exhausted, yet there you are, with more driven worry stirring within. You're caught in a whirlpool of thoughts, feeling lost without a life jacket.

Think of those times when you're trying to sleep but keep wondering, "Did I lock the door? Did I reply to that email?" Staring at the ceiling at 2 AM isn't cool.

So, what's left that actually stops this cycle? **Acknowledge** it. Sounds simple, right? Getting to peace amidst that whirlwind of thoughts is difficult but game-changing.

Instead of letting yourself get chewed up in that cycle of worry-feeding-thinking-feeding-worry, try to pause momentarily. It's easier said than done, but tiny acts add up. Go for tasks matter-of-factly? Taking a break helps. This is where techniques come in that'll nurture your weary mind... Staying aware, taking mind breaks, using guided calming techniques - each step helps you wind down.

Burnout comes on strong 'cause your engine (that's you) opts for eternal anxious thinking. Try to yield to your senses - feel the wind, taste life's simplicity, bask in the moment. Remember, it's not rocket science, right?

Chill out with conscious taps, ease your grey matter - let calming waves lull this roaring beast. Get a proactive nicotine hit (figuratively), take short mindful strolls amidst nature's stress-defying cover. Let the street sounds merge with life's symphony. Watch as clarity and ease cover the detour from those mighty violent cycles, honoring balance and ushering you back into your heart's rhythm, free to defeat the frenzy of anxious-feeding thoughts that had bound you.

How Stress Fuels Overthinking

Ever notice how your **thoughts** go into overdrive when you're stressed? It's like your brain gets stuck in overthinking mode, making **decisions** way harder. Stress doesn't just mess with your feelings; it messes with your thinking too. When you're stressed, simple things turn into complex puzzles. Even choosing what to have for **dinner** can feel like rocket science.

Ongoing stress is like having a foggy brain 24/7. You get easily flustered and can't think straight. This makes picking between options a real headache. We're talking about overanalyzing every little thing, second-guessing yourself non-stop, and feeling trapped in a loop of uncertainty. The more you stress, the tougher it is to break free. Everything becomes a big deal, tasks pile up, and before you know it, you're drowning in your own **thoughts**.

So, what's the deal? How does stress create such chaos in your mind?

Let's chat about **stress hormones**. When you're stressed, your body pumps out hormones like cortisol. These are like your body's alarm bells, meant to help you face immediate dangers. They're great in short bursts, but not so much when they're hanging around long-term.

Cortisol messes with your **brain** more than you might think. It impacts your memory, making it harder to recall stuff. You might walk into a room and completely forget why you're there. With stress hormones flooding your brain, your focus goes out the window, and important tasks slip through the cracks. Even your creativity takes a nosedive. Stress basically hijacks your brain's normal functioning.

Also, high cortisol levels wreak havoc on your **sleep**, causing restless nights and groggy mornings. Lack of shut-eye further clouds your judgment and ability to make decisions. It's like a vicious circle. High stress leads to overthinking, overthinking leads to more stress, and round and round we go.

Here's the scoop — stress, overthinking, and constantly dwelling on problems are all tangled up. When you're stuck overthinking, you waste tons of time going over scenarios in your head, many of which never happen. It's like having a broken record playing the same worries on repeat. This builds stress, which fuels more overthinking.

Ever felt like you can't switch off your brain no matter how hard you try? That's because your mind gets used to this cycle. Your brain creates a habit out of worry, overanalyzing every conversation, action, or choice. Talk about exhausting!

Think about how rough this is on your mental health too. Continuous stress and overthinking keep you on edge. You start feeling jittery, easily irritated, and everything seems like it's falling apart. It's tough to find peace or take a break from your thoughts.

Breaking free means acknowledging this cycle. Recognize when stress is taking over and actively find ways to calm your mind. Sometimes, it's as simple as chatting with a friend, taking a walk, or setting small, manageable tasks.

When you make room for relaxation and clear your **mind**, you give yourself a fighting chance against overthinking. It's all about taking it step by step and finding what works to reclaim your peace.

In Conclusion

In this chapter, you've uncovered how **overthinking** can hijack your mind. By grasping the **triggers** and patterns that fuel overthinking, you're now equipped to handle it better. We've broken it down so you can understand how **emotions** play a role and how to keep them in check.

You've learned about the importance of **self-awareness** in catching your overthinking habits. Common thought patterns like "what-ifs" and "should-haves" are often linked to overthinking. You've also discovered how emotional triggers, such as **stress** and fear, can kickstart a cycle of overthinking.

It's clear now how **anxiety** and overthinking feed off each other, making you feel worse. You've explored the stages of overthinking, from the initial **trigger** to more intense worry.

The **tools** and insights from this chapter can help you act before overthinking spirals out of control. As you apply what you've learned, you'll find it easier to maintain a peaceful and **focused** mind. Remember, you have the control to make a positive difference in how you think and feel every day!

Chapter 3: Foundations of Positive Psychology

Ever wondered why some people seem genuinely **happy**, even in tough times? I often think about the magic behind their smiles and cheerful attitudes. This chapter is all about showing you the secrets to that **spark** in life. You might be curious about what could make you feel that upbeat. Imagine getting to the core of what **positive** thinking can do. I'll guide you through ideas that help boost your **happiness** and overall well-being.

You'll find easy-to-grasp **principles** here and even some surprising comparisons between this and traditional approaches to the mind. This isn't just about feeling good short-term but understanding the **science** behind lasting happiness. Ready to get a peek into how this can change your perspective on everyday life?

By the end, my hope is you'll be itching to apply these ideas. So, let's dive right into uncovering that better you. You're about to embark on a journey that'll shed light on the **foundations** of positive psychology and how they can transform your outlook. From understanding the power of gratitude to exploring the impact of mindfulness, you'll discover a wealth of tools to enhance your **well-being**.

As you delve deeper, you'll learn how to harness your strengths, cultivate resilience, and build meaningful relationships. These aren't just feel-good concepts; they're backed by solid research and real-world applications. You'll see how small shifts in your thinking and behavior can lead to significant improvements in your life satisfaction and personal growth.

So, buckle up and get ready to explore the fascinating world of positive psychology. Who knows? You might just find the key to unlocking your full potential and living your best life.

Introduction to Positive Psychology

Positive psychology is all about **focusing** on what's right with you instead of what's wrong. Think of it as flipping the script. Rather than zeroing in on the negatives – the things that drag you down – positive psychology wants you to spotlight your **strengths**, your joys, and everything that makes you tick. It's about building a life that feels satisfying and worth living.

The aim of positive psychology isn't just to make you happy. It's about improving your overall **well-being** and helping you live your best life. Instead of harping on all the things that could go wrong, it's more about nurturing what makes you feel good and positive.

When you think about psychology, you probably picture therapy, treating mental illness, and stuff like that, right? Regular psychology usually **focuses** on diagnosing and treating disorders to bring someone back up to "normal". The spotlight is often on fixing what's broken. Positive psychology, on the other hand, is about taking what's already good in your life and making it even better. It's like adding sprinkles to an already great ice cream cone.

It's a bit like **gardening**. In regular psychology, you'd remove the weeds, tackle the pests, and fix watering problems that get in the way of your plants growing. But in positive psychology, you're adding nutrients to the soil, giving your garden a little more sunshine, and doing those extra things that really make your plants thrive. It's more about giving that extra oomph rather than just mending the basics.

So, how exactly does this make your everyday life better? Good question! Let's break that down. When using ideas from positive psychology, you're able to shift your **focus**. Instead of ruminating on mistakes or anxieties, you get to amplify the good stuff.

Think about simple daily **practices**. Keeping a gratitude journal – jotting down a few things each day that you're thankful for can really change your outlook. Celebrating little wins, recognizing what you're good at, and connecting more deeply with the people around you can create a powerful positive shift. All those bits and pieces come together to build a more joyful picture.

Suddenly, you're not just going through the motions. You're appreciating what you've achieved, feeling closer to the people around you, finding more reasons to smile each day. This shift brings better emotional **resilience**, stronger relationships, and a generally happier mood. Quite the win-win, don't you think?

In short, positive psychology is like a secret weapon tucked under your arm. It helps you stop overthinking and stressing about all the "what ifs." Instead, you get to live in the "what now" and appreciate what's already great in your life. So, starting today, why not try to shift your focus? Give those positive habits and thoughts a little more space in your mind. You'd be surprised how much of a difference it can make in your daily **happiness**. That's what this whole positive psychology thing is all about.

Key Principles of Positive Psychology

Let's talk about **flourishing**. It's like when a plant blooms beautifully in the perfect environment, but with people. In positive psychology, flourishing means living your best life – full well-being, being happy, and feeling good about yourself and everything around you. When you're flourishing, you're in a groove, moving through life's challenges with a smile. You're soaking in good vibes, connecting deeply with friends, and bouncing back even when things get tough. It's about **thriving**, positivity, and embracing life's ups and downs with a can-do attitude.

Now, let's connect this to **character strengths** and virtues. These are like the ingredients you need to create that thriving life we just talked about. Positive psychology puts a lot of emphasis on this idea, saying that when you tap into your unique abilities and virtuous traits, you feel awesome. Not in a braggy way, but in a true-to-yourself kind of sense. Imagine cooking a meal and tossing in all your favorite spices - that's what character strengths do for your mindset. They pump you up, help you tackle problems, and make you proud of what you bring to the table. Kindness, bravery, creativity - these bulldoze stress and make you feel on top of things.

Speaking of tough times, let's move on to **positive emotions**. You know that warm fuzzy feeling when something really cool happens? Well, those good vibes aren't just momentary distractions. They have this neat trick of sticking around and being the army that fights back against stress and negativity. When you fill your life with joy, gratitude, and optimism, you actually stock up on mental 'snacks' that sustain you during challenging times. Think of positive emotions as your mental toolkit. Regularly experiencing happiness and contentment keeps you ready for whatever life throws your way, making it easier to shake off setbacks and keep smiling through it all. That glossary of good feelings isn't just filler; it's the main gig in building a sturdy and stress-free mental fortress.

In tying it all together, consider each principle as a puzzle piece in the larger picture of a happy, well-rounded life. **Flourishing** sets the stage, **character strengths** and virtues are your starting lineup, and **positive emotions** keep the ball rolling. This blend of key points demonstrates something pretty vibrant: positive psychology isn't just a picker-upper; it's a solid foundation for handling life's roller coaster. So, by understanding and applying these principles, you're setting yourself up for a smoother, richer ride.

The Science of Happiness and Well-being

Have you ever wondered why some days you just feel **fantastic**, while others, not so much? Well, it might surprise you, but it has a lot to do with how your brain is wired. Your brain is like a circuit board, designed to keep you safe and secure. It's always on the lookout for anything that might stress you out or make you unhappy. That's its job. But here's the kicker: this same wiring can also mess with your happiness.

Your brain has pathways, and these pathways become strong when you use them a lot. If you keep thinking bad thoughts, those pathways get stronger. But if you start thinking good thoughts, you can actually carve out new pathways. It's like building a road in your brain. **Positive** thoughts pave the way to more happiness, while negative ones... not so much. It's pretty cool how much control you have over this!

Moving on from the gear and gadgets in your brain, let's talk about what makes you truly **satisfied** and fulfilled in life. You know that feeling when you accomplish something meaningful, or when you're surrounded by loved ones? That's not just random joy; it's real satisfaction! True fulfillment comes from things like building good **relationships**, achieving personal goals, and having a sense of purpose.

Imagine your life is a garden. The seeds you plant and how you take care of them determine what kind of garden you'll have. If you plant seeds of good relationships, kind deeds, and personal achievements, you'll grow a garden full of satisfaction. It takes effort, sure. And it takes time. But it's worth it. You can't just expect happiness to pop up like a weed—it's more like a beautiful flower you nurture.

Now, here's something interesting. Have you noticed how, over time, you tend to get used to the good things in life? It's like that

34

euphoric feeling you get when you first get a new phone, and then, meh, it's just your phone after a while. It's called **hedonic adaptation**. Your brain gets used to happiness, which makes you want more, and sometimes different things, to stay that happy.

Imagine eating your favorite chocolate bar every day. At some point, it stops feeling like a treat and more like a habit. Your brain is built to adapt – it gets used to good things quickly. The concept isn't bad; it keeps you striving for new goals and dreams. But it also means that long-term **happiness** doesn't come from material things or passing pleasures.

In conclusion, you can't just rely on external stuff to make you happy. You need to find joy in simple, everyday moments, create meaningful connections, and give yourself **challenges** that lead to growth. So, if you want to be truly happy, it's time to work on those brain pathways, focus on what truly satisfies you, and understand that getting used to good things isn't necessarily bad. It just means you need to be more **mindful**, more often.

Positive Psychology vs. Traditional Psychology

When you look at **positive psychology**, it really shakes up how you think about mental health. Instead of zeroing in on what's wrong or broken, this approach turns the spotlight on what's working right. So, rather than harping on about problems, positive psychology asks what your **strengths** are. What makes you tick? It's like tending a garden, where you nurture the healthy plants instead of just yanking out the weeds. This shift can be super empowering. Instead of seeing you as a bundle of issues to fix, positive psychology sees you as someone with amazing **capabilities** to develop.

For instance, traditional psychology might dig into your anxiety and try to uncover all the reasons you're feeling jittery. But positive psychology would ask what you're good at and how you can use that to bring more balance and **happiness** into your life. It's all about flipping that lens from problems to potential.

This doesn't mean we're tossing traditional methods out the window. Actually, positive psychology plays really well with them. Think of it like adding tools to your toolbox—more ways to help you out. Traditional techniques can pinpoint the root causes of your issues. Positive psychology can then swoop in to build on your strengths and help you grow even more. They're like two peas in a pod.

Picture this: you're **struggling** with depression. Traditional therapy might kick off by unpacking the origins—maybe it's past trauma or chemical imbalances. Positive psychology would look at what you enjoy or excel at, nudging you to engage more with those aspects to lift your mood. The two approaches can tag-team like a dynamic duo for your overall well-being.

Yet, it's not all sunshine and rainbows. Positive psychology does have its fair share of **critics**. Some folks think it's too Pollyanna-ish, almost to the point of sweeping real problems under the rug. There's a worry it could make you feel like you have to be chipper 24/7, which isn't exactly realistic. Life's not just about feeling good but also about weathering the storms.

Another bone of contention is that some believe positive psychology doesn't dive deep enough. It might just skim the surface without really getting to the heart of the matter. By focusing mainly on strengths and positive aspects, it sometimes risks downplaying serious mental health issues. Imagine someone telling you to just look on the bright side when you're dealing with deep-seated trauma—it might not cut the mustard for everyone.

As nifty as positive psychology is, it's got to be balanced with traditional methods for a full picture of mental health care. No one-size-fits-all solution exists for everyone's needs. Both approaches, when used in **tandem**, can offer a more holistic and genuine path to **well-being**.

In Conclusion

This chapter has opened a new door to **positive psychology**, teaching you ways to brighten your mind and uplift your feelings. It's shown you easy and effective strategies to **boost** your happiness and well-being. Remember these golden nuggets from the chapter:

You've seen what the core ideas and **goals** of positive psychology are, and how it stands out from more typical psychological approaches. You've learned why **positive emotions** should be part of your daily life, the importance of character strengths and virtues, and what makes **happiness** a part of a long, satisfying life.

These nuggets are simple but **powerful tools**. Use them to bring more joy into your daily life. Every small step you take toward **positive thinking** makes a huge difference. Keep going, and you'll feel the change!

Remember, it's all about **cultivating** a brighter outlook. By focusing on the good stuff and nurturing your strengths, you're paving the way for a more fulfilling life. It's not about ignoring the bad times, but rather about building resilience and finding the silver linings.

So, go ahead and put these ideas into practice. **Embrace** the power of positivity and watch as it transforms your world. You've got this!

Chapter 4: Mindset Shifts for Overthinking

Ever felt like your mind just won't stop **racing**? I get it. I've been there too. This chapter is all about shaking things up in your thinking. Switching gears.

Imagine if you could **change** the way you look at your thoughts. You, breaking free from those pesky **cycles**. This chapter's your chance to do exactly that. Forget long-winded lectures; we're diving straight into practical stuff.

Think about **growing** the way you see challenges. Being kinder to yourself when things don't go right. Ever talked down to yourself? Yeah, been there. We'll **challenge** that. Turn it around. Positive vibes and all.

And guess what? There's a handy **exercise** at the end to put all this into practice. You've got this. Make a start. Here's your chance to feel **lighter** up there. Dive in. **Transform** with me.

Developing a Growth Mindset

A **growth mindset** can be a game-changer for you. When you believe you can improve and get better at things, that hope keeps you from getting bogged down in overthinking. Instead of fretting over every little slip-up, you're more likely to zero in on what you've learned and how you can up your game next time. It's like shifting your focus from what's going wrong to what's still possible.

So, how does this forward-looking approach cut down on overthinking? Usually, when you're stuck in an overthinking rut, you're replaying the same problems on loop in your head. "How did I mess up?" "What should I have done differently?" But with a growth mindset, you start asking more helpful questions like, "What can I **learn** from this?" or "What steps can I take to improve?" This focus on learning and growth yanks you out of a cycle of negative thoughts and plops you into a pattern of positive action. Overthinking thrives on uncertainty and doubt, but a growth mindset brings clarity and confidence. A clear mind doesn't stew over past mistakes; it plans for future wins.

Now, let's connect this idea to something crucial: **self-talk**. The way you chat with yourself has a massive impact on how you feel and act. If you believe you can't change or get better, your self-talk is likely full of putdowns and criticism. "I'm just not good at this," or "I'll never be smart enough." This negative chatter fuels overthinking, making mountains out of molehills. But when you start believing you can grow, everything changes.

A growth mindset flips that negative self-talk into something more productive. Instead of self-doubt, your inner voice starts saying things like, "I didn't nail it this time, but I can try a different approach." Or, "I just need more practice." You switch from tearing yourself down to building yourself up. This shift can be empowering and liberating, giving you the mental space to step back from overthinking and take constructive steps instead. Your focus moves from problem-obsessing to solution-seeking.

Here's a nifty trick that can help reinforce this shift in perspective: the "yet" trick. It's super simple but very effective. Whenever you catch yourself saying you can't do something, just add "yet" to the end of your sentence. "I can't solve this problem," becomes, "I can't solve this problem... yet." That tiny word adds a world of possibility. Suddenly, it's not that you can't do something at all—it's just that you haven't figured it out *yet*. It turns a closed door into an open one.

The idea here is to see **challenges** and setbacks as temporary, rather than permanent conditions. You start to look at hurdles as part of the journey, rather than as end points. This can drastically change your relationship with overthinking. Instead of seeing a bump in the road as a sign of failure, you view it as a learning opportunity. "I haven't figured out the answer yet" invites curiosity and exploration, while "I can't do this" invites defeat and worry.

So, keeping a growth mindset does more than just help you stay positive. It sets a powerful foundation that stops overthinking in its tracks. When you believe you can always get better, you're not as likely to get trapped in loops of doubt and worry. You shift from a state of anxiety to one of proactive **problem-solving**. And let me tell you, this mental switch makes a world of difference. You go from feeling stuck to feeling capable. From anxious to hopeful.

Remember, **developing** a growth mindset is a journey. It takes practice and patience. But the payoff? It's huge. You'll find yourself less caught up in overthinking and more focused on growing, learning, and moving forward. So give it a shot. Your future self will thank you for it.

Practicing Self-Compassion

Let's chat about being **kind** to yourself. You know, sometimes you're your own worst enemy. You can be so harsh and critical, especially when you overthink. You replay your mistakes, worry about what-ifs, and just can't let go. But what if you treated yourself like you'd treat a friend? Sounds pretty sweet, right?

Being kind to yourself can make a world of difference. Instead of all that harsh self-talk, imagine saying, "It's okay, you did your best." Being self-compassionate can be a game-changer by countering all that negative noise in your head. It's like swapping out a mean coach for a supportive one.

Now, let's dig into what self-kindness actually means. Turns out, it's not just about cutting yourself some slack. There are three parts to this concept:

First, there's self-kindness. This is just being gentle with yourself. Instead of being your toughest critic, try being your biggest cheerleader. Talk to yourself like you would to a bestie who's going through a rough patch. This takes the sting out of those anxious thoughts and makes them easier to handle.

Next, there's common humanity. Overthinking can make you feel like you're on an island, the only one struggling. By recognizing that everyone messes up and has tough days, you can feel more connected and less alone. Remember, it's human to make mistakes and worry, and you're not the odd one out in this experience.

Last but not least is **mindfulness**. Don't freak out, it's not as complicated as it sounds. Mindfulness is just about being aware of your feelings and accepting them without blowing them out of proportion. So, instead of getting sucked into a vortex of worries, you can stay grounded. Just acknowledging your thoughts without judgment can take away a lot of their power.

Together, these three parts work wonders on reducing **anxiety**. Think of it like a well-balanced recipe for feeling better about yourself.

But hey, maybe you're wondering how to make this self-kindness thing a habit. One super easy technique is the "self-kindness break." This can be your go-to when **stress** levels go through the roof. It's pretty straightforward, too.

When you're feeling overwhelmed, take a pause. Find a quiet spot and sit comfortably. Close your eyes and take a few deep breaths. Imagine inhaling calm and exhaling stress. Next, remind yourself that it's okay to feel what you're feeling. You might say something like, "This is tough, but I'm doing my best."

Then, remind yourself of common humanity. Think of all the other people who may be feeling the same way right now. It helps to normalize your experience.

Finally, say some kind words to yourself. Imagine you're talking to a friend who needs support. Say things like, "I deserve kindness," or "I'm going to be okay." This little exercise can shift your **mindset** quickly and make those spiraling thoughts simmer down.

So, that's the deal with practicing self-compassion. It's not about pretending everything is perfect. It's about being kinder to yourself so you can manage your **thoughts** without letting them run your life. Being kind to yourself might feel strange at first, but stick with it. You'll soon find it makes navigating tough times a lot more manageable.

Enough heavy stuff for now. Give that "self-kindness break" a shot next time you're feeling overwhelmed. You—not just anyone, you—deserve it.

Challenging Negative Self-Talk

Let's face it, you've got this little voice in your head that sometimes turns against you. **Spotting** when your self-talk gets all bad and harsh on you is one of the keys to stopping those overthinking loop-de-loops. Imagine your brain is a radio, and sometimes it tunes into a station full of doubts and negativity. **Catching** yourself when your mind starts playing these negative tracks can be a huge game-changer. Instead of just listening, start asking questions. "Is this thought actually true?" or "Would I say this to a friend?" By questioning these bad thoughts, you can start to weaken their grip.

Breaking the **habit** of overthinking begins here. When you catch a rotten thought, hold it up to the light. Does it make sense? Is it helping you, or just bringing you down? Often, you'll realize it's more like a noisy neighbor than a truth-teller. The more you practice, the easier it gets to spot these untrue, unhelpful thoughts. It's about training your brain to recognize these pesky intruders and not let them squat in your head.

Now, about changing how you **think** to knock down anxiety and stress. Once you've spotted those nasty thoughts, you've got to flip the script. Picture your brain carrying a heavy load of stress – every negative thought is like an extra brick you're lugging around. But if you think in a kind and positive way, each bit of positivity lightens the load. Try to replace negative thoughts with something more balanced, or even totally shift them to something upbeat. Simple tweaks – like thinking, "I messed up," to "Everyone makes mistakes, and I can learn from this" – can make a big difference.

Lowering **stress** is tricky because your mind loves to hang onto unpleasant scenarios. Still, with practice, you can teach yourself to let go. I've been there: stuck replaying a bad comment or mucking up some task at work. Frankly, it's draining. By swapping out those persistent, stress-inducing thoughts, you're freeing up mental space to focus on solutions or just to relax. Remember, it's a marathon, not a sprint. Every positive thought is a small step towards a less anxious mind.

Now for a cool trick: the "thought stopping" **strategy**. When you catch yourself spiraling into negative thoughts, try this: say "Stop!" either out loud or in your head. (Personally, I prefer louder when I'm alone – makes it feel more real.) Then quickly shift your attention to something totally different. It might feel a bit jarring at first, but it intercepts the bad thought pattern and stops it in its tracks.

After saying "Stop!", give your brain something nice to chew on – a favorite **memory**, a song, or even a quick task that keeps you busy. It's kind of like changing the channel when you dislike what's on TV. The moment can't fix everything, but it's a powerful short-circuit for negative spirals.

If combining catching, changing, and stopping feels like learning a sport, you're right. Like any skill, it takes **practice**. With time, you get better, and overthinking starts to lose its grip, letting you breathe easier.

So next time self-talk goes wild or anxiety creeps in, remember these steps. Start with recognizing and questioning those thorny thoughts, shift your mindset from negativity to balance or positivity, and use thought-stopping to cut off the endless worry cycle. All these together can give your mind the peace and calmness it truly deserves.

Reframing Negative Thoughts

Have you ever looked at a situation and felt only bad things snowball? Sometimes, just **tweaking** the way you see things can turn those negative thoughts into something a bit more balanced. It's like wearing a new pair of glasses.

Imagine you've got a mountain of tasks at hand, and you're thinking, "I'll never get this done" or "Why am I so bad at this?" That's the pessimism taking over. But changing your **mindset** could be as simple as asking, "What's one small step I can take now?" You're not ignoring the tasks, just seeing them in a lighter way. Suddenly, it's not about failure, but about taking one step. You'll feel a lot better.

Changing how you think about situations doesn't just affect your thoughts. It helps you manage how you feel too. Once, I was really worried about a presentation. I kept telling myself I was going to mess it up. But someone said, "Why don't you think about it as sharing what you know with others?" It was a small shift, but my jitters went away, or at least they shrunk.

Let's look at another way to rethink things. You're angry because someone cut you off in traffic. The **anger** bubbles inside. But what can help is asking, "Why might they have done that?" Maybe they're rushing to an emergency. You're not excusing their behavior, just rethinking it a bit—this way, anger has room to cool down.

Now, we've talked about how changing thoughts can change feelings. Let's get into the technique that makes this happen, called "**reframing**." It's like this... instead of seeing a rainstorm as ruining your picnic, think of it as a chance to have a fun indoor adventure. Easier said than done, sure, but it works with a little practice.

When something bugging you comes up, ask yourself, "Is there another way to look at this?" Here's a trick: Imagine you're giving advice to a friend who's dealing with the same stuff you are. You'd probably be kinder to them than you are to yourself, right? Apply that same kindness to your situation.

You can also **challenge** your negative thoughts directly. Let's say you messed up a task. Instead of thinking, "I'm a failure," ask, "What did I learn from this?" Turning mistakes into lessons changes everything—now you've got bad moments sprinkled with meaning.

The cool thing about reframing is once you get into it, it becomes second nature. You'll start catching and shifting negative thoughts more often without even trying. Think of it as a small **habit** that can make a big difference over time.

Changing your **perspective** might seem like a tiny tweak, but it packs a punch in battling negative thoughts. Little shifts in the way you see the world can bring balance, help you control your emotions, and, with tools like reframing, offer new ways to tackle whatever life throws your way. And before you know it, you'll feel much lighter, more at ease, taking everything as it comes and finding better ways to dodge **negativity**.

Practical Exercise: Positive Self-Talk Script

Imagine you're sitting there, and a **bad thought** creeps up on you like it always does. This happens to everyone. You're not alone in this at all. Grab a pen or open a notes app. Now, let's go through this together. Yes, really take part in this—we're fixing the messy mind.

Think of a common bad thought you often have. It might be something like, "I'm not good enough at my job," or "I'm always messing things up." It doesn't have to be huge; just something that pops up regularly and eats at you. Write it down.

Alright, let's get to the **feeling**. What do you feel when that thought comes up? Maybe it's frustration, maybe it's sadness, or even a mix of things you can't quite put your finger on. We don't have to pinpoint it exactly, but just try to capture that heavy vibe. Note it down next to that bad thought.

Next, you're putting on your detective hat. **Question** that bad thought by looking for proof for and against it. If you think you're bad at your job, ask yourself, "What's the concrete evidence that I'm bad at my job?" Maybe there was that one mistake, sure, but what about the times you did something right? List those out too. Okay, it's hard. But stick with it—find a balance between the critical you and the kinder you.

Once you've got some info to work with, it's time for a switch. Make a positive, but **realistic statement**. We're not talking about over-the-top cheerleading here. If you're stuck on "I'm bad at my job", try something like, "I'm still learning and everyone makes mistakes," or "I've done good work before, and I can do it again." Write that down.

Practice saying this positive statement every day for a week. Now, this sounds cheesy, I know. But it really works. Look in the mirror.

Whisper it when brushing your teeth. Sneak it into your before-bed thoughts. You need to repeat it. It's like training a muscle—consistent effort changes everything over time.

After that week, pause for a moment and look back on how your **feelings** and actions shifted with this new self-talk. Did you catch yourself feeling a bit lighter, or maybe you approached work with a tad more confidence? Maybe your body isn't as tense, or you felt a bit braver in a meeting. Notice those changes, however small.

This process isn't magic. It's work, but work that truly feels rewarding. All this effort to switch a hurtful thought to a strong, helpful one can eventually become second nature. These steps create a **habit**—a mindset thief turned guardian of better thoughts.

Accept that unlearning old circuits and building new ones won't be immediate. It's like tending to a garden: pulling weeds, nurturing growth, celebrating every small bloom. So, whenever a bad thought shows up again, you've got your positive script ready.

Okay, that's it. You're now equipped to take on your pesky thoughts with some serious constructive attitude. Life gets clearer. The confusion gets quieter. Let's switch up that self-talk consistently, keep going. It's **worth** it.

Conclusion

This chapter was packed with **strategies** for overcoming overthinking by teaching you to shift your **mindset**. Implementing these methods can help bring a sense of calm and control back to your thoughts and overall mental **well-being**. Here are the key takeaways:

You've seen how adopting a **growth** mindset can help lessen your tendency to overthink things. Believing that you can improve yourself can reduce negative self-talk and make you more

optimistic. The power of the "yet" technique helps you reframe challenges by thinking of them as temporary setbacks.

Practicing **self-compassion** can counter harsh self-criticism and reduce anxiety. By identifying and questioning your negative thoughts, you can disrupt the patterns of overthinking.

By using these **techniques**, you can transform your thinking and manage stress more effectively. Keep applying what you've learned and watch the positive changes unfold. Push forward, learn from your experiences, and remember to practice kindness toward yourself every step of the way. Your mind is your most important asset—take care of it!

Chapter 5: Immediate Strategies to Stop Overthinking

Ever wish you could just hit the pause button on your **brain**? I know the feeling all too well. You're constantly caught up in **thoughts**, running in circles. This chapter is your go-to guide for taming that mental chaos. Imagine gaining **control** over those spiraling thoughts. Exciting, right?

I'll walk you through easy-to-follow **strategies**. You'll try the STOP Technique and grounding exercises that promise quick wins. There's also a really neat 5-4-3-2-1 technique which is a lifesaver when things get too noisy upstairs. You won't be a passive reader here – nope, you'll actually engage with a 5-minute overthinking **interrupter**.

Trust me, by the end of this chapter, you'll have some new **tricks** up your sleeve to hush those relentless thoughts. Ready to take **charge**? This might just spark a whole new way of looking at things for you. Can't wait for you to **dive** in.

The STOP Technique

You know that feeling when your mind just won't stop **spinning**, like a hamster on a wheel? Sometimes you just need a quick **break**. Well, the STOP technique can help with that. It's a sort of mental hack to give you that pause button your mind craves when it can't stop overthinking.

Why do you need this kind of break, you ask? Psychologically, breaking thought patterns is like hitting the reset button. Your brain tends to go down the same road it always does, creating ruts, like on a muddy path. It leads to overthinking and, honestly, more **stress**. But if you can stop that cycle, even for a moment, you interrupt the loop. It gives you just enough space to regain control and calm down.

Alright, here's how the STOP technique works. It's super simple and easy to remember:

• Stop: First, you stop whatever you're doing. Literally, stop. It's like when you're running and suddenly come to a halt. This physical action alone can create a jolt in your thoughts. Like turning a noisy machine off, notice the sudden stillness.

• Take a Breath: Next, take a breath. A deep one. Inhale through your nose, hold it for a few seconds, and then exhale slowly through your mouth. Breathing is magical—you might not think about it, but it's your body's way of saying, "Calm down, we got this."

• Observe: Then, observe. What's happening around you? What are you feeling? It's like looking at your thoughts from a distance. Instead of being tangled up in them, you're just noticing them, like clouds passing by.

• Proceed: Finally, proceed. Move on with your day, but do it with whatever you've learned from those earlier steps. Maybe you realize there's no point in stressing about something you can't change. Or you notice you were overthinking something trivial. Now, you have the option to act based on what you've observed.

So, why is it helpful to break the cycle? Simple: every time you change your thought pattern, you create new **pathways**—a little like rerouting traffic. Doing this interrupts your brain's tendency to go down the same unhelpful roads, giving you a fresh perspective.

Don't think this technique is magic, though. It takes **practice**, like anything worth mastering. But once you get the hang of it, you'll notice you aren't caught in those endless spirals so much.

Imagine yourself standing at a crossroads with a backpack full of your **worries**. When you STOP, you actually unzip the backpack, take a breath, see which items are weighing you down, and decide to only carry what's necessary as you move forward.

So, next time you find yourself falling into a loop of overthinking, try this simple technique. It's like giving your mind a time-out—an act of kindness to yourself. Remember, your thoughts can be heavy, but you don't have to carry them all the time.

In the end, being able to pause and catch a breath can make all the difference. This isn't just about managing bad thoughts but about giving yourself a **break**—because, frankly, you deserve it. The STOP technique isn't about stopping your life; it's about taking a moment to truly **live** it.

Grounding Exercises

Ever feel like you're **stuck** in your head, going around and around with no end in sight? Grounding exercises can change the game by moving your **focus** from those thoughts to what's actually in front of you. It's like anchoring yourself to the moment, pulling you out of those overwhelming whirlwinds.

Start by paying attention to where you are right now. Notice the chair you're sitting on or the **sounds** around you. This gets your mind to drop the constant loop of thoughts. Pretty straightforward, right? When you zero in on the here and now, those anxious, wandering thoughts don't stand a chance. It's almost like you can switch off the never-ending chatter.

But there's more to it. Grounding isn't just about snapping back to reality. Using your **senses** to ground yourself benefits the brain in some cool ways. Imagine you're piecing together a puzzle. Each sense – touch, taste, smell, sound, sight – is like a piece of that puzzle. When you're using them all, your brain gets fully engaged with the world around you. It's like taking a breather from running and just walking for a bit.

Catching a whiff of something nice or hearing a bird chirp can trigger feelings of calm. Our senses can influence our thoughts more than we realize. When multiple senses get involved, it's like telling your brain to chill out. It sends **signals** through your nervous system that help calm your mind and reduce stress.

Shifting gears now, there's this nifty trick called the "5-4-3-2-1" sensory awareness **exercise**. It's a surefire method for getting grounded, fast.

Here's how it goes:

• List five things you can see. They don't have to be extraordinary – maybe it's the lamp on your desk, or the mug you forgot to wash.

• Find four things you can touch. The texture of your shirt, the cold surface of your phone, or even the carpet beneath your feet.

• Listen for three things you can hear. It might be the hum of your AC, distant chatter, or even your own breathing.

• Think of two things you can smell. This bit can be tricky, but there's always something – maybe the scent of soap on your hands or that cup of coffee brewing in the kitchen.

• Identify one thing you can taste. It could be the remnants of your last meal or just the fresh mintiness of your toothpaste.

By the end of this exercise, you're almost guaranteed to feel more centered. It's a brilliant **strategy** for when you're getting really pulled into your anxious thoughts.

Just like that, whether it's grounding by taking in your surroundings or doing the "5-4-3-2-1" exercise, these small but mighty practices are a real **asset** in calming an overthinking mind. Give them a try next time you catch yourself spiraling. It might just be the little shift you need.

Thought Diffusion Methods

Ever tried to take a step back and just **watch** your thoughts float by? Thought diffusion might sound like some high-tech term, but it's actually super simple. It's all about finding some space between you and those annoying thoughts that pop into your head.

Imagine this: You're driving and suddenly feel a wave of panic about work piling up. Thought diffusion helps you realize that these thoughts are just like clouds passing in the sky—not permanent, not all-consuming. When you practice this, you're able to see thoughts as just thoughts—nothing more, nothing less. It creates room to **breathe**.

But what exactly is this thought diffusion? It's also known as cognitive defusion. Big word alert! But don't sweat it, it's actually pretty straightforward. Cognitive defusion is about letting go of the idea that your thoughts are super important and need to be acted upon. Thoughts can be tricky—they often feel like literal truths. You know that feeling: "If I think I'm going to fail, I must be set to fail."

When practicing cognitive defusion, you **acknowledge** that thoughts don't have to dictate your reality. They're not powerful truths, just your brain doing its thing. It's like carrying a heavy backpack and then realizing, "Hey, I can put this down whenever I want."

Now, let's get into a practical tool—the "leaves on a stream" **visualization**. This trick is a neat way to practice thought diffusion. Here's how it goes: Close your eyes, take a few deep breaths, and imagine you're sitting by a flowing stream. There are leaves gently floating along the water. Each time a thought pops up, just place it on a leaf and watch it drift away. If it comes back, no big deal, just let it float away again.

Why does this work? Well, it's like giving your thoughts a pathway to exit. Instead of letting them circle around in your head, you watch them leave. It's soothing and helps break that intensity thoughts can hold over you. Sometimes, I imagine those leaves getting stuck on rocks, but gently, they always find their way again and move along.

Picture it like this—your thoughts are not you. They come and go, just like leaves on that stream. You're the **observer**, not the struggler swimming against the current.

Incorporating these little practices into your day can lead to big changes. Next time you're having one of those moments filled with spiraling thoughts, take a seat by your imaginary stream. It's a bit of you-time and mental **decluttering**.

So, thought diffusion might feel like a tiny shift, yet it packs a punch. By taking that mental step back and watching your thoughts float by, you keep a friendly distance. Cognitive defusion reminds you thoughts aren't reality, and little tricks like "leaves on a stream" turn an overwhelming mental storm into a peaceful day outside.

Give it a shot! See those leaves drift and realize you've got this— the ability to let go, **breathe**, and let thoughts flow by like a lazy stream on a sunny afternoon.

The 5-4-3-2-1 Technique

When you're stuck in a loop of **overthinking**, it feels like you're trapped in your own head. One way to snap back to reality is the 5-4-3-2-1 technique. It's super simple and quick, helping you break up those relentless cycles of unnecessary thoughts.

Picture this: you've been **stewing** over something for hours. Maybe it's a conversation you had, or a mistake you made. Your mind refuses to let it go, replaying the same scenario again and again. That's where the 5-4-3-2-1 technique steps in. This method uses your **senses** to ground you in the present moment. It basically forces you to observe what's around you right now instead of what's bouncing around in your brain. You see, focusing on tangible things pulls your mind away from the endless cycle of worry.

Think about it, your senses are directly tied to what's happening right now. Not yesterday, not tomorrow. There's real power in paying attention to your senses because they're directly feeding your brain with info about your surroundings. Using them to break overthinking kinda tricks your mind into exiting that loop.

Alright, let's walk through the exact steps of how this **technique** works:

Start with five things you can see. Go ahead, look around. Find five things you can see right now. They don't have to be interesting or different. It could be your coffee mug, the carpet, a poster on the wall. Just point them out in your mind. Making your mind actively search for these items puts your focus on your environment, right this minute.

Next, four things you can touch. This one's all about feeling. What are four things you can physically touch? It might be the smooth surface of your table, the fabric of your shirt, or the pages of a book. Use your hands, feel the textures. Notice how doing this pulls you back into experiencing the present physically.

Oh, and before we move on, don't rush. Take your time to really feel those objects. It's a kind of **mindfulness** that ensures you're just here, interacting with real stuff.

Then, three things you can hear. Turn up your listening skills a bit. Identify three sounds around you. It could be the hum of the fridge, the ticking of a clock, or birds outside. Listen carefully. This step makes you pay attention to the environment through your ears and distracts your mind from overthinking.

After that, two things you can smell. Now engage your nose. Nothing elaborate; you don't need to smell perfume or something fancy. It could be the scent of your soap or even fresh air coming from an open window.

Finally, one thing you can taste. Move to taste. It might be a bit challenging if you're not eating, but maybe you can still taste a lingering flavor or even grab a small snack to complete this step. You'll be amazed at how focusing on this 'tiny' sense shifts your thinking gears.

Doing all these things? It's like an off switch for your racing mind. By the time you've identified all five senses, your focus has moved far, far away from whatever you were overthinking about.

There you've got it—engaging your **senses**. Trying these steps anytime you're stuck in a mind-loop will help. Just give this technique a shot, and see how it feels to **anchor** yourself in the present.

Practical Exercise: 5-Minute Overthinking Interrupter

Ever feel like your **mind** is a washing machine stuck in spin cycle? When you're overthinking, it's like getting tangled in a messy web of your own thoughts. But here's a neat trick that takes just five minutes to interrupt that cycle. It's simple, and it starts with setting a timer.

Grab your phone and set a **timer** for five minutes. This small step marks the beginning of calming the tornado in your head. Why a timer? It's like telling your brain, "Hey, we're doing this for just a short bit, then we're done." Knowing it's only five minutes can make you actually want to give it a shot.

Start by taking three deep **breaths**. Don't rush. Just inhale slowly and let the air fill up your lungs. Exhale. Notice how it feels. Cool air going in, maybe warm air coming out. This simple focus on breathing can steer your mind away from the chaos, planting you right back into the moment. It's like hitting the pause button on your scattered thoughts.

Next, look around and name five things you can **see**. Maybe there's a book, a lamp, a picture on the wall, your phone, or even a tree outside the window. By doing this, you're forcing your brain to switch channels, from the internal chatter to the external reality. It grounds you, making your surroundings more real than the spiraling worries.

Now onto touch. Find four things you can **touch** and describe what they feel like. Grab that cozy blanket, the smooth surface of your table, or the rough texture of your jeans. Notice each sensation. The soft cushioning of a pillow, the cool ceramic of a coffee mug. Describing these things slows your mind, engaging it in a more soothing, tactile experience.

What do you hear? Pause and listen for three different **sounds** around you. Maybe it's the hum of a fan, birds chirping outside, or faint music in the background. Each sound pulls you further away from overthinking and draws your attention to the world beyond your thoughts. It's no magic trick, just focusing on what's actually present around you.

And scents...let's not skip those. Notice two **smells** in the air. Maybe it's laundry detergent in your clothes or freshly brewed coffee. Take them in, no matter how subtle. Identifying smells can be surprisingly calming. It engages a different part of your brain, one that doesn't entertain worry and stress. Plus, it's kinda nice to just smell stuff.

Finally, think about one thing you can **taste**—or remember a flavor. Maybe you've got a piece of gum handy, or perhaps you bring to mind the taste of your favorite meal. Doesn't really matter. What's important is that thinking about taste can serve as one more anchor to the present, helping you steer clear of overthinking land.

By the time your timer rings, you've walked through five senses and sealed yourself right into the present moment. These small, mindful actions can fight the stronghold of overthinking. And trust me, they add up. Interrupting the overthinking cycle becomes second nature with practice, and you'll find it easier to drift into moments of calm.

After you try it, claim this time each day—even just once. It's like building a mental muscle. See these five minutes as a micro break from your overactive mind. Trying this whenever you feel the swirl starting can make all the difference. So, why not give it a go?

Conclusion

This chapter gives you immediate **strategies** to stop overthinking and stay **calm**. By learning practical **exercises** and understanding the principles behind them, you'll be better equipped to manage **anxiety** and negative thoughts whenever they pop up. The techniques mentioned are simple yet effective ways to shift your **focus** and reduce stress.

In this chapter, you've seen:

• How the STOP technique can offer a quick break from overthinking

• The psychological reasons why interrupting thought patterns is helpful

• The importance of grounding exercises to shift your focus to external sensations

• The concept of thought diffusion to create distance from intrusive thoughts

• Practical exercises like the 5-4-3-2-1 technique to interrupt cycles of overthinking

Remember, applying these **strategies** every day will help you manage thoughts and **stress** better. The more you practice, the more natural it'll become. Take these tools and use them whenever you feel overwhelmed. You've got this!

Chapter 6: Cognitive Restructuring Techniques

Have you ever wondered why you let **bad thoughts** mess with your head? Seriously, it's like you're your own worst enemy sometimes. In this chapter, get ready 'cause I'm gonna guide you through a few **tricks** that could completely change how you see your mind's **chatter**.

So, think about that moment when you catch yourself **spiraling** into a bad mood. We all do it. But what if you could hit pause and actually **rethink** those automatic, destructive thoughts? I'll show you how.

It's gonna be fun—like fixing up a tangled mess into something neat and **balanced**. You won't just read about it; you'll see it in action, feel it shift your **perspective**. By the end of this chapter, you'll see your thoughts in a whole new light.

Ready to **rewire** that mind of yours? Let's get into it!

Identifying Cognitive Distortions

Recognizing cognitive **distortions** can really help you break those overthinking patterns. It's like putting on new glasses and suddenly seeing things clearly. When you spot these distortions, you start to see how your mind is tricking you into seeing things worse than they are.

One of the most common cognitive distortions is "All or Nothing Thinking." You know, when you see everything as either black or white. For instance, if you make one little mistake at work, you might think you're a total failure. This type of **thinking** can really mess with your mood and make you feel stressed. But understanding that life is full of grays, not just blacks and whites, can help you feel more balanced.

Another one is "Overgeneralization." This is when you take a single event and apply it to everything in your life. Like if one bad thing happens, you think it'll always happen. So, you screwed up that presentation? Doesn't mean you're doomed to always suck at public speaking. It's just one event.

Then there's "Mental Filtering." This is when you focus on one bad thing and ignore all the good stuff. Maybe someone gave you some negative **feedback**, and now it feels like the whole project was a bust, even though there were loads of positive remarks. It's like looking at life through a pair of dark-tinted glasses.

How about "Discounting the Positive"? Well, this is when you downplay good things that happen to you. So, you aced a test and think, "Oh, it was just luck" instead of giving yourself credit for studying hard. This steals your **confidence** and fuels more overthinking.

Knowing about these common distortions is eye-opening, right? But simply knowing them isn't enough. You've gotta learn how to spot them in action.

This is where the "Distortion Detective" technique comes in. Think of yourself as a detective on a mission to find irrational thoughts. When you have a thought that makes you upset or stressed, pause. Ask yourself, "Is this really true?" Check if you're falling into any cognitive distortion. If you can identify and name the distortion, you've already weakened its power over you.

Start by writing down your **thoughts** when you feel off. Maybe you're worried about a speech. Write down exactly what you're thinking. I'll bet some distortion will come up. Is it All or Nothing Thinking? Are you filtering out the good stuff and only seeing the possibility of messing it up? Once you've spotted the distortion, challenge it. Ask, "What evidence do I have for my fear? Is there another way to look at it?"

Now you're a distortion detective, and it's normal to slip up while you're learning this. It's a **skill** you build over time. With practice, this technique helps in reducing overthinking and getting a clearer brain space. So, next time negative thoughts flood in, you'll be ready.

In wrapping up, identifying cognitive distortions can be a real game-changer. Keeping an eye out for those pesky mind tricks helps you stop overthinking and lets you focus on more positive and realistic thoughts. The distortion detective technique? Your new best friend. Regularly finding and confronting these distortions shifts your **view** and reduces your **stress** levels. You're on your way to a calmer, clearer mind.

The ABC Model of Thoughts and Emotions

Ever wonder why you feel a certain way in a situation? It's like having a secret **user manual** for your mind. The ABC Model, by Albert Ellis, offers that glimpse. It helps break down how you can figure out how your thoughts mess with your emotions, connecting the dots in ways that might surprise you.

You might catch yourself thinking, "It's all chaos!" when you overthink things, but hang on—there's an order to this madness. The ABC Model shows you're not going nuts; your thoughts, beliefs, and reactions have a method to the madness. So hang tight, and let's break this down one piece at a time.

Picture this: You have an event, something happens, and that's what we call an "**Activating Event**." It's like a trigger that sparks off a chain of thoughts. So you have this event, and right after, comes the "**Belief**." This is what you tell yourself about the event. And finally, based on this belief, there's the "**Consequence**," which is how you feel and what you do next. See? Simple as ABC.

Take a spilled coffee as an example. If your belief is, "I'm so careless," the consequence might be feeling crummy all day. But change that belief to "Mistakes happen," and your consequence is much different—it's just a hassle, not a day-ruiner. Cool, right?

Okay, this is great and all, but how do you use this when you overthink? Here's where it gets handy. When you're in one of those **spirals**, you can use the ABC Model to dissect the situation. So you start by identifying the Activating Event. What exactly is bothering you?

Let's say, your boss emails you about an unfinished task right before the end of the day. That's your event. Next, what's the Belief? Maybe you start thinking, "I'm terrible at my job." Now, check the Consequence. You're stressed and you're already itching to send a hundred emails to fix everything. It's clear: the entire loop is exhaustively playing its part in your mental gig.

So now, let's switch gears and hit that belief stage. Question your logic. Is it possible that the belief is not the whole truth? Maybe you think, "I had a busy day, and it's just one task." How does that change the consequence? Your **stress** dips, and you're not racing in a panicked frenzy.

Alright, here's where this model shines in guiding you through your overthinking tangent. Once you get familiar with using the ABC Model, you can start checking your thoughts anytime they go spirally. One crumb on the floor doesn't ruin the whole cookie, right?

The beauty of this is, you start catching yourself mid-spiral. You're like, "Oh! That's an activating event. What dumb belief am I spinning now?" Just a tiny self-check-in works wonders—it's disturbingly effective.

But don't expect magic overnight. Use it day by day, snack-sized. Going through emails? Spinning out? Boom, ABC it. A rude comment from a stranger? ABC on that. Piece by piece, notice how your reactions align with new beliefs. Challenge yourself often— old habits stick hard.

In life, things happen that throw wrenches in your peace. But consider having this ABC Model as if it's a **toolkit** in your pocket. Whenever you seem stuck in a loop of overthinking, you're trained to check off events and beliefs causing your reactions. This new way of thinking could just be your relief switch.

Next time you find yourself caught in those nagging thoughts, remember the ABCs. Shift your beliefs, change your consequences, and see stress melt away, bit by bit. No need for handling every worry that comes your way; just equip your mind to understand and swap narratives. And all at once, it might make this habit of **overthinking** finally melt away. Cool beans, huh?

Evidence-Based Thought Challenging

Feeling **trapped** in your mind because of worrying and stressing isn't great. You've been there. But sometimes, breaking down these thoughts isn't so hardcore. A practical way to check your thoughts is gathering **proof**. Why believe every nagging thought your brain throws at you? Seeing is believing, right?

Imagine you've got this big **presentation**, and your mind decides to tell you you'll mess it up. Hold on—is there any solid reason behind that thought? Instead of taking what your brain tells you at face value, dig a little. Look back and see if you've given any horrible presentations in the past. Maybe not. In fact, you likely did just fine, or maybe even nailed it! So, why would this time be any different?

Seeing things **objectively** matters more than you think. It's like stepping back and seeing the full picture instead of zooming in on the tiniest details. Imagine you're looking at a big painting. When you focus only on one small corner, you miss out on the beauty of the whole thing. Treat your thoughts the same way. Too close, and they seem disastrous, but a bit of distance, and they're not so terrifying.

Moving from proof to seeing things objectively, let's say your mind says no one likes you. That's heavy. But take a step back—what's the real scene around that? You're jumpy about your friends not replying instantly. Are they busy? Did they act warmly the last time you met? Probably, yes. **Thoughts** can be sneaky, zooming in on negatives and blurring out the positives. But facts don't lie. Looking at the entire situation eases off anxious and stressed feelings a bit.

One cool way to hit this head-on is using an "**evidence** log." Consider it your personal thought-scoring book. When a lousy thought pops up, jot it down. Next, gather proof for and against that thought. The more you scribble, the clearer things get.

Say you're freaked about a meeting at work. Your mind screams you're unprepared. Write that down. For this thought, jot notes showing you've prepared all week. You might see there are hardly any valid blunders from past meetings. This log helps dial things down and see reality.

Seems like a big chore at first, but soon it becomes second nature. Having those few honest scribbles often lighten the mental load. Try it the next time mental stresses cloud your mind. Let me give you an example from last week. I was so fixated on a small **critique** from a peer that it almost felt like the world was ending. Writing this down and digging proof pulled me right out from drowning in those thoughts.

And like that—three solid ways to chisel away unnecessary **stress**. From collecting proof, seeing the bigger picture, and keeping an evidence log, your mind can stop racing. Each of these steps equips you to put up a decent challenge against that grenade of overthinking your mind loves to throw.

Creating Balanced Thoughts

Coming up with **balanced** thoughts can really cut down on that all-or-nothing thinking. You know, the kind where if one little thing goes wrong, the whole day is ruined? It's like thinking in black and white, with no shades of gray. When you learn to balance your thoughts, it's like adding a full spectrum of colors to your mind.

For example, instead of thinking "I failed that test, so I'm a complete failure," you might think, "I didn't do well on that test, but it doesn't mean I'm a failure. I can do better next time." See the difference? You're bringing in a more nuanced view that takes the pressure off and makes it easier to deal with setbacks.

To create this habit, start by catching yourself when you're having these absolute thoughts. Ask yourself: Is there more to the story? Maybe there are other factors you haven't considered. This simple act can put you on the path to more balanced thinking.

So, give it a shot. When you have a negative thought, counter it with another perspective. Maybe it's as simple as, "I'm having a tough day, but it doesn't mean the whole week is bad." This way, you're training your brain to see the middle ground rather than swinging from one extreme to another.

Now, how does being mentally **flexible** help? Well, imagine your thoughts are like trees in a windstorm. If they're rigid, they snap. But if they bend, they survive. Mental flexibility is about being able to adjust your thoughts and expectations when new information comes in. It helps manage overthinking because you're not stuck on one fixed idea.

Being flexible in your thinking isn't about abandoning your core beliefs. It's more about being open to adjusting them. Maybe today, you think you're awful at presentations. But with a bit of practice and some positive reinforcement, that belief can change. You're not fixed; your mind is capable of adapting.

And when you're flexible, it's easier to stop spiraling into worry. For instance, if something unexpected comes up, instead of panicking and thinking your plans are ruined, you adapt. You think, "Okay, this isn't what I expected, but I can work with it." You become more **resilient**, less likely to get stuck in endless loops of what-ifs and worst-case scenarios.

Here's the cool part: you can practice **flexibility** with simple exercises. Try thinking of multiple ways to solve a problem rather than sticking to just one solution. Or challenge yourself to see if there's a different way to look at a situation that's been bothering you. It's like mental yoga – the more you do it, the more flexible your mind becomes.

This leads us to the "both-and" technique. This technique can help you come up with more detailed thought patterns. Instead of thinking in "either-or" terms, you think in a way that holds two truths at once. For example, "I can be disappointed by my performance and still be proud of my effort."

Using "both-and" changes everything. It allows for a more **nuanced** view, which in turn makes your thoughts richer and more balanced. When you catch yourself thinking in absolutes like, "I can either be successful or I can be happy," try this: "I can both be successful and work on my happiness."

Think of it as a way to add layers to your thoughts, like adding depth to a painting. You're not just thinking in flat colors anymore. Each time you practice "both-and," you disrupt old habits of rigid thinking and introduce more balanced and realistic **perceptions**.

So here's a little exercise: the next time you find yourself caught in a loop, try "both-and." You might find it brings a whole new **perspective** – it's surprising how this small shift can make a world of difference in reducing **overthinking**.

Practical Exercise: Thought Record Worksheet

Ever get caught in a **whirlwind** of your own thoughts? It's like a snowball effect, right? One small thing happens, and before you know it, your mind's taken you to some worst-case scenario. Here's a way to stop that from happening. Let's dive into the "thought record worksheet" technique, which can really help you **break** the cycle.

First, think of a situation that made you start overthinking. Picture a **trigger** that caused that overthinking spiral. Maybe you received an unexpected email from your boss late at night. Suddenly, you're convinced you're in trouble, your job's on the line, and the world's crashing down.

Next, grab a piece of paper and jot down all those initial **thoughts**. What were you thinking? Maybe it went something like, "I'm going to get fired," "I can't handle this," or "Everything is going wrong." These are your automatic thoughts – the ones that pop up right away without much prompting.

Now, take a look at those thoughts. How do they make you feel? Rate each **emotion** on a scale from 0 to 10 on how intense it feels. This helps you get a sense of which thoughts are stirring up the heaviest emotions. You might find that "I'm going to get fired" ranks a solid 8 or 9, giving you that tight feeling in your chest.

After that, it's time to spot cognitive **distortions**. These are like glitches in your thinking patterns. Maybe you're catastrophizing, magnifying the situation way out of proportion, or engaging in some serious black-and-white thinking - like believing one small mistake means ultimate failure.

Time to play detective! For each automatic thought, find **evidence** for and against it. If you thought, "I'm going to get fired," what supports this? Maybe nothing, besides you getting that email. Now, what's the evidence against it? Perhaps you've received positive feedback recently, or maybe the email didn't say anything alarming.

Based on the evidence, come up with a more balanced, alternative **thought**. Instead of thinking, "I'm going to get fired," maybe you come up with "One email doesn't mean I'm in trouble. I can wait until I have more information." The idea is to find a middle ground, something more realistic that fits the actual evidence.

Finally, look at your new, balanced thought and re-rate your emotions. How intense are they now? Chances are, they've dialed down quite a bit. Maybe that fear drops from a 9 to a 4. Not erased, but **manageable**. This shows that you actually have power over your thoughts and feelings.

Doing this exercise regularly can help you train your brain to stop overthinking before it spirals out of control. It's about taking control, one thought at a time.

In Conclusion

This chapter has shown you different ways of **thinking** to help stop overthinking and stay **calm**. You've learned about some common thinking **mistakes** and how to fix them, used a special model to understand your **feelings**, and practiced finding proof to challenge your thoughts. Let's quickly sum it up, and don't worry, it's easier than you think!

You've seen how spotting mind tricks can help you think clearly, and you've explored common types of thinking errors and their **impact**. The ABC model has shown you how your thoughts and feelings link up. You've also learned to gather **evidence** to test if anxious thoughts are true or not, and create balanced thoughts that aren't too extreme, but more fair.

Great work! Remember, every time you notice one of those sneaky overthinking **patterns**, take a breath and try these **tools**. You're already on your way to a calmer and happier mind!

Chapter 7: Emotional Regulation Strategies

Ever wonder what it'd be like to have a **remote control** for your feelings? Well, in this chapter, you'll find just that. With me as your guide, you're about to take an enlightening stroll through the remarkable world of **emotional regulation**. Imagine having the tools to recognize what you're feeling, like you've just unlocked a secret code to your own mind.

As I share these insights, think about the moments you've felt **overwhelmed**, not knowing how to handle your own emotional storms. You're not alone. We all ride the same rollercoaster of moods and feelings. But what if you could direct that ride?

So, gear up! Together, we'll get to grips with **understanding** and labeling emotions, express them effectively, and use nifty **strategies** like the opposite action technique. By the end, you'll walk away with a personal **toolkit** for handling whatever life throws your way. This chapter? It's your **game-changer**.

You're about to dive into a world where you can take charge of your emotions, rather than letting them run the show. It's like becoming the director of your own emotional movie. You'll learn how to spot what you're feeling, give it a name, and then decide what to do about it. It's not about suppressing your emotions – it's about riding them like a pro surfer rides waves.

Remember those times when you felt like your feelings were too big to handle? Well, you're about to learn some cool tricks to shrink them down to size. And the best part? These aren't just pie-in-the-sky ideas. They're practical, down-to-earth techniques that you can start using right away.

Understanding Emotional Intelligence

Have you ever felt **overwhelmed** by your emotions? They can spiral out of control, making everything seem worse. That's where being emotionally smart, or having **emotional intelligence**, comes in handy.

Being emotionally smart means you're good at spotting, understanding, and handling your own feelings. It also helps you manage how you react to what others feel. Imagine staying cool when chaos hits, or keeping calm during an argument. Emotional smarts mean fewer moped rants and more level-headed thinking.

Let's dive into the details. Emotional smarts have four key components: knowing your own feelings, **managing** them, understanding others' feelings, and handling relationships properly. Each of these bits plays a crucial role when it comes to overthinking.

Knowing your own feelings sounds pretty basic, right? But you'd be surprised how often we misname or miss them entirely. This isn't about being bad at feelings; it's about labeling them correctly. Feel like you're sinking in quicksand? It may not be pure anger but a mix of frustration and embarrassment.

Then there's managing those feelings. It's tough not to vent all over the place or hide under your blanket. Being emotionally smart means keeping your anger in check, not faking a smile. It's about finding ways to stir yourself out of grumpiness without taking it out on others. Overthinking often crashes here. That repeated inner chat? Learning to pause and **refocus** is key.

Let's bridge this to understanding others' feelings. Imagine knowing why your coworker snaps or spotting your friend's hidden stress. Less guessing what went wrong, more finding real connections. Without this part, you end up doubting yourself and getting stuck in your thoughts.

And then there's the relationship part – handling other people. It couples your skills into strong, thriving connections. You read cues, spot troubles before they blow up, and take proper actions. Fewer **conflicts**, more peace.

Alright, how do you get better at knowing and noticing your feelings? One useful trick is the "emotion wheel." Ever seen it? It's a colorful circle with a magic list of feelings, from simple ones like happy and sad to tricky ones like annoyed or hopeful.

Using this wheel, start naming what you feel. Imagine you're super nervous before a big meeting. Check the wheel – could it be **anxiousness** mixed with excitement? Sometimes putting a label stops feelings from ruling us. Just like that, you peg a feeling before it eats you alive.

But don't just spot them, notice when they come. There's power in saying, "Yeah, I'm feeling kind of anxious." It makes you less of a mess and way more in control.

Wrapping this up helps us circle back to where we began. When you lean into emotional smarts and piece out those four bits – knowing feelings, managing them, cluing into others, and juggling relationships – overthinking takes a backseat. No more mental races or wasted **brainpower** over trivial stuff. Next time, remember, it's about being smart with feelings, not letting them boss you around.

Recognizing and Labeling Emotions

Sometimes emotions can feel like a huge, tangled **mess**. But here's the thing: figuring them out can actually make them less overwhelming. Each **emotion** you experience aims to tell you something. But you can't always understand what it's saying until you take a pause and tune in. Once you identify what you're feeling, it suddenly becomes more manageable.

Picture this: you're swamped with work, dealing with family **problems**, and you feel like you're about to explode. If you sit down and think, "Okay, I'm anxious and a bit angry," you've taken the first step in defusing that bomb. It's like sorting out a drawer full of junk—once you know what's in there, it doesn't seem that full or scary.

Getting to the bottom of what you're feeling can calm the **chaos**. It's about separating emotions from that big jumble in your head and giving them names. Whether it's sadness, frustration, or even joy, naming them helps in shrinking their power over you. So, rather than wrestling with a vague storm, you can say, "Ah, there it is, I'm feeling this and that." And that's pretty empowering.

But there's more to it than just feeling better. Your **brain** actually benefits from this exercise. When you name your emotions, it fires up specific parts of your brain, helping you process everything better. Labeling emotions isn't just some fluffy talk—it's real brain science.

When you're stressed, sometimes your brain does this thing where it sends you into fight-or-flight mode. Labeling your emotions can shut that down. By doing so, you move from being reactive to reflective. High performers in every field talk about this—athletes, leaders, artists. They all use it to keep their **stress** in check and their minds sharp.

Here's a cool tip: if you say your emotions out loud, the effect seems to be even greater. So next time you're stressed out, give it a shot. Say, "I'm feeling overwhelmed," and notice how that simple act can make a big difference. Suddenly, the sky starts to clear, and you can breathe a bit easier. It's like your brain gives a little sigh of relief.

Now that we've covered labeling, let's link those emotions with your physical feelings through the "body scan" method. This one's pretty neat and super practical. The body scan is like checking in with different parts of your body, noticing what's happening, and seeing how they relate to your emotions.

Start by sitting or lying down in a comfy position. Close your eyes if it helps. Imagine scanning your body from top to toe. Notice any tension or weird sensations. Maybe your shoulders are tight, or there's a knot in your stomach. These physical feelings often tell you what your mind might be too busy to recognize.

If you find your jaw clenched, you might be angry. If your chest feels heavy, perhaps sadness is creeping in. It's a great way to really know what's going on inside of you. When you connect the dots between your body and your emotions, **solutions** to your issues become clearer. You might realize you need to cool off or, maybe, you just need a good cry.

Linking physical sensations with emotions can be super enlightening. Not only does it help you understand what's stressing you out, but it also tells you how to handle it. So next time things get crazy, pause and do a quick body scan. That small pause can become your best ally against overwhelming emotions.

Naming emotions and doing a body scan aren't just tricks; they're real techniques to make sense of life's messiness. Recognize what you're feeling, say it out loud, and tune into your body. By doing this, you'll see how much easier it is to navigate through stressful times.

Effective Emotional Expression

You know how sometimes your mind **runs** in circles, like a hamster on a wheel? Too much overthinking can really drag you down. But expressing your emotions in a healthy way can help. It's like releasing steam from a pressure cooker. When you're able to put your **feelings** into words, you stop worrying so much. You don't keep replaying things in your head. Your brain takes a breather, and that gives you mental space to be present and enjoy life.

When you bottle up your emotions, it's like holding a ball underwater. You know it's only a matter of time before it pops back up. Not dealing with your feelings can make them come out in nasty ways later on. Maybe you've noticed that when you don't talk about what's **bugging** you, it builds up. You might snap at someone for no reason or feel really down without knowing why.

But dealing with emotions is different. It's like letting the ball float calmly on the water. You acknowledge it. You accept it. And you find ways to express it, so it doesn't control you. One way to do that is through effective **communication**.

Here's a handy tool: the "I-statement" technique. This method is a simple way to express your feelings without making others feel attacked. You start with "I feel," then say your emotion, the situation, and why. For example, "I feel upset when the kitchen is messy because it makes me feel like no one cares."

Using "I-statements" helps keep the conversation calm and focused on your feelings, instead of blaming the other person. It's like shining a light on your own emotions rather than pointing fingers. This way, you can talk things out without escalating into an **argument**.

For instance, if your friend forgot to call you back and that hurt your feelings, instead of saying, "You never call me back!", you could say, "I feel hurt when you don't return my calls because it makes me think you don't care about our friendship." This method helps keep the focus on how you feel, making the conversation more about finding a solution rather than winning a fight.

Another benefit of "I-statements" is that they make you more self-aware. You start to pay attention to what you're feeling and why. It's like peeling an onion – you get to the core of what's really **bothering** you. It's surprising how often the things that upset us have simple solutions once everyone knows where they stand.

In the end, this technique isn't just about better communication with others. It's also about better understanding yourself. When you can clearly express how you feel, it stops you from overthinking.

Bottling things up only turns simple issues into bigger **problems**, making your mind race even more. But when you deal with your emotions and use tools like "I-statements," you keep things practical and straightforward. This brings you peace and helps you stop dwelling on stuff all the time.

So give this a shot next time you're feeling overwhelmed. Say how you feel. Use "I-statements." See how it changes things for you. Remember, your goal is to keep your emotional ball floating calmly, not holding it underwater.

The Opposite Action Technique

Strong **emotions** can drive you nuts, making you overthink everything and putting you in a bad mood. But what if doing the opposite of what you feel could actually help? Sounds a bit weird, right? This trick works wonders, though.

When **anger** hits, your gut reaction might be to yell or slam doors. Instead, try talking softly or walking it off. You're tricking your brain here. Anger wants to explode; calmness defuses it. Doing the opposite floods your system with different vibes, making those intense feelings lose their grip.

Why does this even work? It boils down to the idea that **actions** can shape how you feel. Think of your brain as a toddler needing distraction. When you're super sad, your brain tells you to curl up in a blanket and avoid people. But if you decide to get out, meet friends, or take a stroll, you're sending new messages to your brain. You start thinking, "Hey, maybe things aren't so bad!"

This switcheroo works because your mind attaches **feelings** to actions. Sitting in the dark makes you focus on sad thoughts. But sunlight or a good conversation pulls your focus away, breaking that bad cycle. It's almost like changing the channel on a scary movie.

Feeling scared? Your typical move might be to avoid what scares you. What if you did the opposite? **Challenge** yourself with small steps. If talking to strangers freaks you out, start by saying hi to a cashier. Positive actions reduce fear bit by bit. Each successful interaction slowly convinces your brain there's nothing to worry about.

When **sadness** hits, you probably feel like avoiding activities or hiding from everyone. Go in the other direction. Get up, go for a walk, or chat with a friend. These opposite-action steps brighten your day because your brain catches up and starts to feel better too.

Now, what about anger? Your instinct might tell you to yell or break something. Try speaking calmly instead or taking a deep breath before reacting. Even better? Go for a quick run or listen to music you love. This shifts anger into something way more manageable.

Then there's **shame**, the one making you run and hide. Face the music instead. Messed up at work? Speak to your boss directly. Ashamed of missteps with a friend? Apologize. The more you confront, the weaker the shame feels.

Anxiety is the jittery one, pushing you to avoid or overprepare. Flip the script. Round up all the ways anxiety tells you to avoid something and actually do it with opposite actions. Prepared way too much for a meeting? Wing some conversation. Avoiding social situations? Volunteer in one. Anxiety melts in the face of actions it wasn't expecting.

Pretty neat, huh? This trick works like a charm. The more you lean into yin when your gut screams yang, the more control you gain over those pesky emotions. Just remember, it's all about taking that first step in the opposite direction.

Practical Exercise: Emotion Regulation Toolkit

Let's kick things off with something super simple but incredibly **important**. Grab a pen and paper and jot down the intense **emotions** you feel most often. It doesn't have to be a long list, just the big ones that pop up a lot. Maybe it's anxiety, sadness, anger, or something else. Keep this list handy because you're gonna use it a lot.

Once you've got your list, it's time to find a physical **grounding** technique for each emotion. Let's take anxiety for instance—it loves to hang out when it's least wanted. A good way to tackle it? Deep **breathing**. Just inhale deeply through your nose, hold it for a few seconds, and exhale slowly through your mouth. Do this a few times and you might feel your heart rate start to chill a bit. Got sadness on your list? Try putting your hand over your heart and take a moment to feel your heartbeat—simple but grounding. Anger might need something a bit more physical, like squeezing a stress ball. This helps bring you back to the present moment and keeps the emotion from running wild.

Next up: positive self-talk. For every emotion, come up with a statement that counters the negativity. Feeling anxious? Try telling yourself, "I've overcome tough stuff before; I can handle this too." Sad? You might say, "It's okay to feel sad, but I know this will pass." Anger? How about, "Getting angry won't solve this." Positive self-talk can seem cheesy at first, but it helps to rewire how you confront these emotions.

Now, let's talk about picking healthy ways to **express** each emotion. Take sadness, for example. Instead of bottling it up, why not try journaling? Just write down everything you're feeling without editing yourself. If you're angry, maybe take up kickboxing, or go for a run. It's amazing how physical activity can siphon off those intense feelings.

Here's a fun and effective one: find opposite **actions** for each emotion. When you feel like withdrawing because you're sad, opt to socialize instead. Feeling anxious and want to run away? Stay put and face it head-on. Anger making you wanna yell? Try breaking into a smile or laughing—it's uncomfortable but it can flip the emotion on its head.

Now it's all about **practice**. Use your toolkit every day and jot down which strategies are working best for you. Maybe you find that deep breathing is your go-to for anxiety, or that you prefer journaling your frustration out more than exercising it away. The key here is to keep at it and track your progress.

Finally, don't forget to tweak. Once a week, take a look at your notes. What's working? What's not? Don't be afraid to make **changes**. Maybe you need a new self-talk phrase or a different grounding technique. It's an evolving toolkit, not set in stone.

Together, these steps create something powerful. A way to manage emotions that can seem unmanageable. Give it time and patience, and you'll see how much it can help you navigate the ups and downs.

In Conclusion

In this chapter, you've picked up a ton about **controlling** your emotions more effectively. We've covered understanding emotional intelligence, **recognizing** and labeling your emotions, **expressing** feelings in a healthy way, and using special techniques to handle intense emotions. Let's quickly recap the key points.

You've discovered that emotional intelligence makes dealing with tough feelings easier. **Knowing** the components of emotional intelligence helps in managing overthinking. Using **tools** like the "emotion wheel" can help you name and understand your feelings better. Properly **identifying** your emotions can make them less overwhelming and prevent them from taking over. The "body scan" technique helps connect your physical sensations with your mental state.

By putting these lessons into practice, you can become emotionally **smarter** and more resilient. Take these **strategies** and apply them in your daily life. Your emotions don't have to run the show. You can manage them, boost your mood, and focus on the positives around you. Keep at it, and you'll be amazed at how much better you can feel!

Chapter 8: Time Management for Overthinkers

Ever found yourself drowning in thoughts, unable to **focus**? That's pretty much how I felt just yesterday. You've got a million ideas buzzing around, but no clear way to tackle them. Feels familiar, right? In this chapter, I'll help you turn that mental **chaos** into smooth sailing.

You've probably heard of **prioritization** techniques. Simple tricks I'll show you that could change how you view important tasks. Got it? And imagine slicing your work into digestible chunks— Pomodoro style! You'll love it.

When it comes to arranging your day, **time blocking** is like having a toolkit right by your side. Plus, Eisenhower's **method** adds a sprinkle of clarity. And before you know it, you'll be carving out a personal **productivity** plan that's tailor-made for your quirks.

Get ready for some real and easy steps to master your **time**. Ready to turn that overthinking mess into efficient **action**? Buckle up, it's time to get things done.

Prioritization Techniques

Got too many things **piling up** on your to-do list? Let's chat about how effective prioritization can save the day. When you've got a hundred things swimming around in your head, it's easy to get stuck in a loop of decision-making. That gets old, fast. It's like your brain just taps out and screams "Enough!" Effective prioritization throws your brain a life preserver. **Decision fatigue** just melts away when you don't have to constantly decide what's next. Think of it as giving your mind a break.

Let's focus on reducing decision fatigue first. Prioritization does wonders here. By laying out what absolutely needs your attention, you remove a lot of stress. Your brain isn't fired up trying to sort what's screaming the loudest for your attention because it already knows. You're no longer sapped just from choosing what to work on next. That saved **energy** can go into knocking stuff out. Less time deciding. More time doing. Imagine having your mental bandwidth freed up. Feels good, right?

On to lowering stress and clearing **mental clutter**. Clutter isn't just physical junk on a desk; it's also all those thoughts bouncing around in your head. Carrying that load is a real drag. Knowing your priorities instantly cuts that down. Each task sorted is like removing a mental post-it note stuck on your brain. It's about replacing chaos with a more relaxing mental landscape. With the madness in check, you don't just feel better - you think better too.

So, let's have a look at a technique to aid in sorting things out, meet the **Eisenhower Matrix**. Named after Dwight D. Eisenhower, it's all about slicing up your tasks into what's important and what's urgent. Sounds basic? Well, it works. Picture a box split into four smaller boxes:

• Urgent and Important

• Important, Not Urgent

• Urgent, Not Important

• Not Urgent, Not Important

First box, urgent and important. This is crisis mode – handle these right away. These tasks set off alarms. Can't put them off, they've got to be dealt with now. Could be deadlines, last-minute issues, really anything that's both critical and time-sensitive.

Now, those important but not urgent wickets go in the second box. These are your long-term goals, planning sessions, projects that mean a lot but won't fall apart if you push them a bit. It's your sweet spot for **strategic thinking**. Things like planning, personal development, stuff that counts but isn't setting your pants on fire right now. Tackling these can really make or break how effectively you're moving long-term.

Next, urgent but not important. Tasks that feel pressing but really provide no value. Things like answering low-priority emails. They demand quick action but in the grand scheme, don't move you closer to your goals. Sometimes these are better off delegated if you can, look at them as interruptions disguised as priorities.

Finally, you've got not urgent and not important. These? Limit or cut as much as possible. Absolute distractions. They aren't helping with stress, or efficiency, or hitting your goals. Great example - excessive social media scrolling or endlessly tweaking a presentation. Just let these go.

Switching gears from theory to action. Use the Eisenhower Matrix on the next pile of tasks and see how freeing it feels. Seriously, knowing what to tackle and what to pass on sharpens your **focus**. It's like giving your brain a tiny vacation each day. From wrestling the never-ending demands to actually seeing daily **progress**. What're you waiting for? Start sorting.

The Pomodoro Technique

Ever feel like you're stuck in a never-ending loop of working and thinking, only to realize you're not really making much **progress**? Structured work intervals can be a game-changer. Have you heard about the Pomodoro Technique? It's this clever little method where you break your work into short, focused **sprints**. Sounds simple, right?

Picture this: you set a timer for 25 minutes, dive into work, and give it your all. When the timer goes off, you take a short break—say, five minutes. This cycle repeats a few times, and believe it or not, it helps you **focus** much better. You're less likely to get caught up in overthinking every little detail.

Those 25-minute sprints, or "Pomodoros," force you to get down to **business**. With a countdown clock ticking, there's less room for distraction or dwelling on unwanted thoughts. You know time's running out, and you've got a task to complete. It's like a race against the clock, and winning feels pretty awesome.

Now, let's talk about breaks. At first glance, frequent breaks might seem counterproductive, right? But hold on—take them, and you'll see it's quite the opposite. Regular breaks keep your mind sharp.

Taking five minutes off every 25 minutes might sound too simple to be effective. But it clears your head. These small pauses help reset your **focus**, prevent mental fatigue, and can even spark creative solutions. Step away from your desk, stretch a bit, or grab a snack. These brief moments give your brain a necessary breather, prepping it for the next Pomodoro.

You know that foggy feeling when your brain's overworked? Taking regular pauses helps clear that away. You're not letting your mind get bogged down with too much clutter. Instead, you're giving it a fresh start, almost like hitting a mental refresh button.

And taking a longer break after a few Pomodoros can work wonders too. Consider having a more extended 15-30 minute break after four cycles. It's like a mini-reward and gives you the **energy** to jump back into another round of focus sprints.

So, what's the Pomodoro Technique all about? Think of it as a handful of easy steps designed to boost **productivity** while keeping anxiety in check. Start by deciding what task you need to work on. Set a timer for 25 minutes. Dive into working. Once that timer dings, take a quick five-minute break.

Finished that Pomodoro? Great! Jot it down. After four Pomodoros, treat yourself to a longer break. Sounds almost too simple, right? But simple is great.

All caught up? Let's wrap this up. Structured work intervals—they work wonders. Breaks—super helpful. Steps—easy and straightforward. This technique packs a punch in beating overthinking and ramping up your **efficiency**. Next time you're facing a mountain of tasks, give the Pomodoro Technique a shot. Who knew tackling overthinking and boosting productivity could be so, well, manageable?

Time Blocking Strategies

Looking for a way to make your day feel less chaotic? Time **blocking** can really help. It's all about planning your day in chunks of time dedicated to specific tasks. When you **schedule** your day, you know exactly what to focus on. No more wondering what to do next. It cuts down on the number of decisions you make and brings order to your routine. Everything finds its place—which can be a huge game-changer for overthinkers.

Let's face it, decision-making **stress** is real. You're constantly thinking about what to do now, then next, then after that. It never stops! But with time blocking, your decisions are made ahead of time. Picture each hour of your day with a label—Morning Routine,

Work Time, Lunch Break, Exercise, Family Time. This routine helps drown out the noise and what-ifs of everyday life, giving you a solid plan—something concrete you can hold onto.

Now, shifting gears to "deep **work**." Ever been so lost in what you're doing that time just flies by? That's deep work—a state of intense focus where you get a ton of meaningful stuff done. It pulls you out of your head and places you in the zone. Overthinking? Out the window. Instead, you're engaged, taking action, and dominating whatever you're working on.

However, achieving this level of **focus** doesn't happen by accident. You've got to set the stage for it, and guess what? Time blocking can help. Visualize chunks of your day blocked off just for this "zone time." It's like creating a bubble—no interruptions, no distractions. Only pure, undiluted focus.

Connecting both ideas, you have a clear picture of what you need to do and time set aside just for that solid, productive work. Let's combine them now into a **strategy** you can use daily.

Time blocking isn't complicated. Start by listing out tasks or activities you need or want to do. Split your day into segments— morning, afternoon, evening. Assign tasks to these segments in a way that makes sense to you. Each task or activity fits snugly into its block of time. Need an example? Your morning might be for waking up, getting ready, and handling basic emails. The afternoon could be for more focused work or big projects. Evening could be for unwinding and spending time with family or friends.

It's like you're painting your day. Each color (or task) goes in its own space on the canvas (your **schedule**). It looks neat, feels orderly, and, guess what, you're in control. Got everything where it should be? Fantastic. Any surprises or new tasks can be slotted into existing days with minimal fuss.

Feedback from those who've tried it? Super positive. They feel less scattered, more grounded. Give it a shot. Start by blocking out a couple of days. Feel how the order brings calmness. With time blocking, your days become less like a messy scattered collage and more like a well-organized art piece. Complete and **satisfying**.

Eisenhower's Method

Ever feel like you're **juggling** too many tasks at once? There are urgent things that need your attention right now, and then there are important things that matter, but not necessarily at this moment. This endless list can steer you onto the overthinking train. What if you could clearly distinguish between what's urgent and what's important? Bingo! Enter Eisenhower's Method.

The **beauty** of Eisenhower's Method lies in its simplicity. You're separating tasks into what's urgent (things screaming for immediate attention) and what's important (things that contribute to long-term goals). This simple shift in how you view tasks can make a world of difference. No more endless loops of what to do next. No more stressing over trivial tasks while the significant ones remain untouched.

Imagine a square divided into four boxes. These boxes are: Urgent and Important, Important but Not Urgent, Urgent but Not Important, and Not Urgent, Not Important. You'd put tasks in these categories based on their nature. Here's how Eisenhower's four sections roll out:

• Urgent and Important: These tasks are crises or **deadlines**. Like when you've got a report due tomorrow and your car breaks down. These need immediate attention and action. It's like juggling with chainsaws—gotta get it done fast, or things could get messy.

• Important but Not Urgent: These are where you want to spend most of your **energy**. Think long-term goals, like planning, learning a new skill, or spending quality time with loved ones. These tasks are essential, shaping your future in a big way, but don't need to happen today or even this week. It's like planting seeds—you may not see the results now, but they're crucial for later.

• Urgent but Not Important: These are interruptions or tasks you don't value deeply but need your attention. Emails, some meetings, or minor requests. They're like speed bumps—slow you down, stall your progress on crucial stuff, but need a quick resolve. Delegating is your best bet here.

• Not Urgent, Not Important: Finally, these are the **time-wasters**—Netflix binges, social media scrolling, or maybe even sorting out already organized drawers. They don't contribute to your goals and can be dropped without any regret. They're like empty calories—fun, but ultimately unfulfilling.

Alright, we've got these boxes. But how do you use them? That's where it's magic for setting task **priorities** effectively.

Start by making a to-do list of everything you think needs doing. Dump it all out, anything that's been crowding your brain, transfer it to paper. Then pick up each task and pop it into one of the four boxes. Found a task that's due and requires all your brain cells intact? That's Urgent and Important. Got a task that's been on your mind but doesn't press you with a deadline? Mark it as Important but Not Urgent. Got it? Great!

Next bit is working with the plan. Aim to conquer Urgent and Important first. They keep the wheels greased, so you're not derailed. But don't let Important but Not Urgent slip through, that's your **growth** zone. If tasks fall under Urgent but Not Important, see if you can delegate them. Trust me, people around you can pitch in! And those Not Urgent & Not Important tasks…well, just toss 'em out or save them if you've got extra time, but don't stress over them.

In the end, using the Eisenhower Method doesn't just bring order to your tasks—it clears the fog in your mind, stops the choke point of overthinking, and brings **peace** to your everyday routine. Instead of drowning in tasks, you're sailing through them. And who doesn't want that?

Practical Exercise: Personal Productivity Plan

Ready to tackle **overthinking** by boosting your productivity? Let's dive in with some clear steps to get you moving in the right direction.

First up, get everything out of your head and onto paper. Think about all the stuff you need to do next week. Everything. Jot down work tasks, home chores, appointments, anything that requires your attention. It might feel overwhelming at first, but that's the point. By laying it all out, you'll start to feel a bit of relief already. This is all about creating order from chaos.

Next, it's time for some sorting magic with the Eisenhower Matrix. This **Matrix** splits tasks into four categories: urgent and important, important but not urgent, urgent but not important, and neither urgent nor important. Go through your list and place each task where it belongs. This visual prioritization will help you see what needs your attention the most and what's just adding to the noise.

Alright, with tasks sorted, let's set up a time-blocked **schedule** for the week. Block specific times for each task category on your calendar. Start with the urgent and important tasks, fitting them into slots early in the day when your energy is high. Next, tackle the important but not urgent tasks. This way, you'll ensure you're working on what matters while still chipping away at the rest. Color-coding these blocks can make the schedule more visually appealing and easier to follow.

To keep **focus** during your work sessions, try the Pomodoro Technique. Work for 25 minutes, fully concentrated, then take a 5-

minute break. Repeat this cycle four times, then take a longer break—maybe 15 or 30 minutes. You'll find that the ticking timer helps keep overthinking at bay since you're zeroed in on short bursts of productivity.

At the end of each day, check your **progress**. See what you've accomplished and what's left to do. This daily check-in helps tweak your plan if needed. Maybe you'll spot a task that's dragging on, which can be rescheduled. Or you might identify time slots that need adjusting for better productivity.

Consider which **strategies** have helped the most in cutting down on overthinking. Reflect on parts of the day when your mind felt calmer and more focused. Did time-blocking give you peace of mind? Did focusing during Pomodoro sessions reduce mental distraction?

After your weekly run, fine-tune your personal **productivity** plan. Incorporate what you've learned about your working style and adjust your tasks and schedule accordingly. This way, each week becomes more streamlined and less overwhelming.

In no time, you'll find a rhythm that suits you. The more control you gain over your tasks, the less your mind will race about what hasn't been done. And that's the ultimate goal—a calmer, more organized way of handling your week, freeing up mental space for peace and positivity. Keep it going, and you'll soon recognize the power of structured **planning** in minimizing overthinking and boosting your peace of mind.

In Conclusion

In this chapter, you've learned about ways to **manage** time better and keep away from **overthinking**. These methods are straightforward, and if you remember to use them, they'll be super helpful in your daily life. Here's what you've seen:

You've discovered that effective **prioritization** helps in cutting down decision fatigue and limiting overthinking. Having clear priorities can greatly reduce **stress** and keep your mind free of mental clutter. You've also learned about the "Eisenhower Matrix," which helps you classify tasks based on their importance and urgency.

The **Pomodoro** Technique, with its structured work intervals, can boost your focus and minimize overthinking. Time **blocking** offers you a better sense of control over your day, lowering stress from decision-making.

Taking these lessons and putting them into **practice** can make a big difference in your life. So start prioritizing, take frequent breaks, schedule your tasks, and aim for a more organized routine. Do this, and you'll find your mind feeling much clearer and calmer. Keep at it!

Remember, these **strategies** are meant to make your life easier, not add more pressure. So don't stress if you can't implement everything at once. Start small, be consistent, and you'll see improvements in no time. You've got this!

Chapter 9: Stress Reduction Techniques

Ever wonder why you're always **stressed** out? You could probably use a break. This chapter will guide you through simple yet effective **techniques** that'll make a huge difference in handling stress.

Imagine being able to **relax** your muscles and calm your mind anytime you want. It's easier than you might think. Maybe you've heard about some **breathing** methods but never tried them. You might be surprised how even a few minutes of the right kind of breathing can make you feel like a new person.

Ever thought about talking yourself into **calmness**? Sounds funny, right? But trust me, it's not. Plus, you'll figure out how to face those little stress **triggers** in your life and stop them from bugging you too much. By the end, you'll have a daily **routine** that fits easily into your lifestyle. Ready to feel more **relaxed** and in control? Let's dive in.

You'll learn how to:

• Use deep breathing exercises to instantly calm yourself

• Practice progressive muscle relaxation for full-body tension release

• Employ positive self-talk to boost your mood and confidence

• Identify and manage your personal stress triggers

• Create a sustainable stress-reduction routine that works for you

So, are you ready to kick stress to the curb and start living your best, most relaxed life? Great! Let's get started on your journey to a calmer, happier you.

Progressive Muscle Relaxation

Have you ever noticed how physically relaxing can make you feel more mentally calm? It's true. When your **body** is at ease, your **mind** can follow suit. Think about times when you had a relaxing massage or spent a few minutes stretching. You probably felt like your brain took a mini-vacation, too. It works because **stress** and muscle tightness are like best buddies—they usually hang out together. Tense muscles are often a sign that your mind is under pressure, and loosening them up can signal to your brain that it's safe to chill out.

Let's talk more about this whole muscle tightness thing. When you're stressed, your muscles might clench up without you even realizing it. You know those times your shoulders are up to your ears or your jaw feels stiff? It's no coincidence. The mind and body are connected like that. Stress causes your sympathetic nervous system to go into overdrive, and muscles tense up as a response. This isn't just annoying—it can keep you feeling stressed out longer. Weird loop, right? So breaking that loop by relaxing your muscles can make your mind stop freaking out so much.

Here's where Progressive Muscle **Relaxation** (PMR) comes in. It's a method that involves tensing and then relaxing different muscle groups across your body. By doing this, you get to notice what **tension** and relaxation feel like, making it easier to spot when you're tense and make a conscious decision to relax.

Now, how do you actually do PMR? It's simple and you can do it anywhere. You might want to get comfortable in a quiet spot to start. The process involves a few basic steps:

• Get Cozy: Find a comfy chair or lie down.

• Breathe Deeply: Take a few deep breaths...in through your nose, out through your mouth. Give your body the signal to start winding down.

• Start With Your Feet: Curl your toes tight—like you're picking up something with them. Hold for about five seconds. Then release and feel those muscles loosen up. Ahh...

• Work Up To Your Legs: Now move up to your calves. Flex them hard for a few seconds, then let go. Feel the difference?

• Move To Your Thighs: Repeat the tightening, holding, and releasing with your thighs.

• Time For The Tummy: Squeeze those abs tight and hold. Let go and breathe easy.

• Don't Forget The Hands: Clench your fists, hold for a few seconds, then stretch out your fingers.

• Focus On Shoulders And Neck: Push your shoulders up toward your ears. Hold, and then release. Let them drop naturally.

• Face Last: Scrunch your face up like a bulldog, hold, and then relax.

By walking through these steps, from your feet all the way up to your face, you're teaching your body how to switch off tension in stages.

Practicing PMR can help you pinpoint where you're holding **stress**. If it feels like this is too detailed to remember right away, it's okay to jot it down on a little card or phone note to guide you. Eventually, you'll start doing it naturally, and the **tension** will melt away quicker each time.

Diaphragmatic Breathing Exercises

Controlled breathing can work wonders for **reducing** anxiety. You know those moments when your mind just won't shut off? Your thoughts race. Your heart pounds. It feels like you're stuck on this never-ending hamster wheel of worry. But, just by focusing on your breath, you can seriously chill out and clear your mind.

When you breathe deeply from your **diaphragm**, it sends a chill-out message to your brain. Think of it like flipping a switch. Your nervous system gets the memo to slow down, calming both your mind and body. Those shallow breaths some people take? They do the opposite. They make you feel all jittery and on edge. Deep breathing, though, tells your body everything's okay.

Deep breathing is basically sound **science**. Your nervous system has two parts: the sympathetic (fight or flight) and the parasympathetic (rest and digest). When you're stressed out, the sympathetic takes over, making your heart race and your muscles tense. But, breathing deeply switches control to the parasympathetic. It's like hitting the brakes in a car. Your body eases up, tension melts away, and you feel a sense of calm.

Here's where things get really cool. The "4-7-8" breathing **trick**. Super easy. Super effective. It works like magic.

Start by exhaling completely. Now, inhale through your nose for a count of 4. Hold that breath for a count of 7. Then, exhale slowly through your mouth for a count of 8. Repeat this cycle about four times. It might seem kind of simple, but trust me—it works. By the time you're done, you'll feel like you've hit a reset button.

As you practice the "4-7-8" technique more often, it becomes like second nature. You'll find you're able to stay calmer, even in situations that used to make you feel **stressed**.

Seeing these techniques come alive in your daily life can be a game-changer. Imagine being stuck in traffic, about to lose it. Instead of flipping out, try the 4-7-8 trick. Or before an important meeting when your nerves are through the roof, a few rounds can ground you and clear your mind to focus.

Using diaphragmatic breathing daily isn't just about handling crisis moments, though. It's all about teaching your body to stay **relaxed** over time. You're retraining your brain to better handle anything that gets thrown your way.

So, knowing how controlled breathing cuts **anxiety**, what deep breathing does to your nervous system, and the 4-7-8 trick puts powerful tools in your hands to handle stress. These breathing basics can seem minor, but their effects stack up, leading to a calmer, more focused, and **stress-free** you.

Autogenic Training

Ever felt so **stressed** that your brain just won't shut up? That's where autogenic training comes in. It's like hitting the reset button on your mind and body. This self-help **relaxation** technique can really chill you out. Seriously, it's like **meditation** but with a twist. It helps you reach deep relaxation and clear your mind of all that clutter.

Autogenic training works by using self-suggestion to calm your thoughts. Imagine telling your body to relax, and it actually listens. That's the magic here. You repeat specific phrases to yourself while focusing on body sensations, like warmth and heaviness. Over time, this **practice** helps lower stress and hush all that overthinking.

Think of it as coaching your brain to chill out, one step at a time. You'll need to find a quiet spot where you won't be interrupted. Get comfy by sitting or lying down, closing your eyes to avoid distractions. Then, breathe deeply: inhale slowly, hold for a count, and exhale. Repeat until you feel more centered.

Here's where the fun part starts—self-suggestion. Let me show you how. Picture this basic script:

• "My right arm is heavy": Say this to yourself repeatedly. Focus on the sensation in your arm, feeling it get heavier.

• "My right arm is warm": Next, tell yourself this. Imagine a warm, soothing flood through your arm.

• Continue this for your left arm, legs, and other body parts: Yep, your whole body gets in on the action.

These phrases might sound simple, but stick with it—the magic happens over time. The key is **repetition** and belief. Doing this regularly can help your body learn to relax on cue, which is especially handy when stress hits hard. Like having a personal escape hatch in your mind.

You're probably wondering how skipping through phases of self-suggestion can impact your day-to-day life. Autogenic training doesn't just relax you, it conditions you to respond differently to stress. Over time, you get better at turning the volume down on all that mind chatter. It's like teaching yourself to flip a switch when things get overwhelming.

This is huge for overcoming **overthinking**. Imagine cutting off the endless loop of worries before it even starts. By regularly practicing these simple scripts, you get a better handle on stressful situations, making them less likely to spiral out of control. It's basically a mental lifehack.

But how does this self-suggestion stuff actually work? It taps into your parasympathetic nervous system, the part of your body responsible for rest and relaxation. By suggesting feelings of warmth and heaviness, you're signaling this system to kick in. It's like telling a snoozing cat it's okay to stretch out and purr. Once your body gets the hint, it sends signals back to your brain, helping to calm your thoughts too.

These little relaxation scripts may sound trivial, but they pack a punch. Making this a part of your daily **routine** can lead to major improvements in how you handle stress. Imagine feeling more in control, less frazzled, and more centered.

So go ahead, give autogenic **training** a whirl. It may feel weird at first, but stick with it. You'll soon find those moments of calm seeping into your busy life, giving you a much-needed break from the chaos. And really, who couldn't use a bit more peace and quiet?

The 4 A's of Stress Management

Ever felt like **stress** is running the show? Well, you're not alone. Having a framework can give you a structured way to tackle things head-on rather than letting them run wild. That's where the 4 A's come in handy. They stand for Avoid, Change, Adjust, and Accept. Let's walk through each one and see how it can help you **manage** stress better.

Avoid

First up is Avoid. Sometimes the easiest way to deal with stress is to simply step away from the things causing it. If certain people or situations are driving you nuts, it's okay to give them the chop. You can, for example, learn to say "no" more often. You don't have to be a people-pleaser all the time. It's about creating **boundaries**. Picture a fence around your mental space where only good stuff gets in. If there's a bunch of traffic and it stresses you out, maybe take a different route. Cut out the things that don't serve you. It's not about running away, but about steering clear of unnecessary bumps on your road to peace.

So how do you use it? Say your job is stressing you out. Could you delegate some tasks or reduce your workload temporarily? Or maybe you have a friend who constantly whines and brings you down. Being honest and taking a break from them could save you a lot of headaches. Small changes like these mean less energy wasted on stress.

Now, once you've figured out what to avoid, you might sense a bit of room to breathe. This makes way for the next step: Change.

Change

Sometimes, steering clear isn't enough, and you need to take things head-on. Change is about actively making alterations. You can't always avoid stress, but you certainly can change how you deal with it. Think about the way you **communicate** your needs or how you manage time. Need some practical methods? Begin by looking at what you can alter in your environment to make it stress-free. A messy workspace can become neat, or a chaotic schedule can become something more organized.

An example might make this clearer. Imagine you're always late. Tweak your routine so you get more breathing room in your schedule. Set a bunch of smaller tasks earlier in the day. This not only helps manage your workload but leaves you space to unwind. Notice the difference it makes when you have some control over what happens around you? Tweaking small bits here and there can have a huge payoff on how much stress rolls your way.

Okay, now we're making some progress with Avoiding and Changing. Still, sometimes you can't avoid the stressors, nor change them enough to eliminate the hassle. That's where Adjust steps up.

Adjust

You dodged some stress and changed some situations. But what about the stuff you can't move around? That's where you need to adjust your **expectations**. It's about reshaping your perspective. Maybe your workload isn't something you can lessen, but your approach towards it can make a world of difference. Are you a perfectionist? Perhaps "good enough" is perfectly fine sometimes.

As an example, let's say you're stuck in a stressful family situation you can't avoid or fix. Adjusting could be focusing on what you can control and reminding yourself that it's okay to not have everything go perfectly. It's giving yourself grace when things fall short. Change what's outside when you can, and tweak what's inside when you can't. Mindset shifts can cause stress to lose its grip on you.

So far, we've dodged, switched up, and shifted our outlook on stress. Yet some situations remain stubbornly beyond our powers to duck or fix. That's when you need to call on Accept.

Accept

Here's the chill factor. **Acceptance**. Some things you can't avoid or change, and aggressively trying to alter them just creates more stress. Sometimes, choosing to accept a situation as it is can free you up. It's about letting go of that fruitless battle against the waves. Picture surfing instead of swimming against the current.

When's it useful? Imagine you're dealing with unexpected outcomes, like waiting endlessly at a doctor's office. You can't change the wait, nor the reality of why you're there in the first place. But accepting the situation while finding ways to stay calm (a book or some music) controls your emotional response. Acceptance doesn't mean giving up; it means acknowledging reality so you can focus on where you can make a difference.

With the 4 A's — Avoid, Change, Adjust, and Accept — you've got **options**. Not every solution fits every problem, but knowing these tools can help you do more than just react to stress. It lets you have a game plan and that is a giant step in calming your mind and relieving **stress**.

Practical Exercise: Daily Stress Relief Routine

Ever feel like your **brain's** running a mile a minute and you just can't catch a break? Well, here's a simple **routine** to help you chill out and recharge. Let's dive into these steps, starting with something easy but effective.

Belly Breathing: Spend just 5 minutes breathing deep into your belly. Breathe in deeply through your nose, filling your lungs and letting your stomach puff out, then breathe out slowly through your mouth. This kind of breathing signals your body to relax and lets you focus on simply being in the moment. You might even be surprised at how **calming** it is to take these few minutes just to breathe.

Next up is a Body Scan. It's a quick survey of your body to see where you might be holding tension. Close your eyes and start from your head, moving down to your toes. Notice any tight or sore spots. Maybe your shoulders feel bunched up, or your back is stiff. Just becoming aware of these tensions can make a difference and prepare you for the next step.

Getting into Progressive Muscle **Relaxation** is the third part. This one's a bit more active than the body scan. For about 10 minutes, you're going to tense and then relax different muscle groups. Start with your toes, curl them tightly for a few seconds, then let go. Move on to your legs, tighten your calves, then release. Work your way up through your body until you've hit all the main muscle groups. This can really help release the tensions you found during the body scan and leave your muscles feeling more relaxed.

Now, it's time to get into a positive headspace with some Positive Self-Talk. This step is about switching up the script in your brain. If you're stressed, your thoughts tend to spiral negatively. So, find some positive things to say to yourself. Simple phrases like, "I can handle this," or "I'm doing my best," can go a long way. Reflecting on your **strengths** and achievements can also provide a calming effect and keep your stress in check.

Picking One Stressor to Apply the 4 A's framework transforms your stress into something more manageable. The 4 A's are Avoid, Alter, Adapt, and Accept. Identify one thing that's stressing you out. Can you avoid it, like by saying no to new tasks? Or maybe you can alter the situation, change how you approach it? Adapting might mean adjusting your standards or expectations. Lastly, sometimes you just have to accept it and move on. This strategy makes your **stress** manageable and actionable.

Next, you wrap things up with two minutes of Gratitude. Think about what you're thankful for. It can be something right in front of you, like a sunny day, or something more personal, like friends or family. **Gratitude** shifts your mindset from what's stressing you out to what's good in your life. It's a nice way to end your routine on a positive note.

Now that you've gone through each step, it's time to check your Stress Levels. Think about where you started. Felt tight, anxious, or frazzled? And now, how do you feel? More relaxed? Calmer? Reflecting on this comparison can help you see the **benefits** of these techniques and motivate you to keep up with the routine.

And there you have it—your daily stress relief routine. Try incorporating this into your daily schedule and see how it changes not just your day, but your overall outlook.

In Conclusion

This chapter has armed you with some **powerful** techniques to tackle stress and curb overthinking. By putting these methods into practice, you'll be on your way to a **calmer** mind and better stress management in your daily life. Let's do a quick rundown of what you've learned:

Progressive Muscle Relaxation helps you connect physical relaxation with mental calmness, putting the brakes on that **overthinking** cycle. Once you get the hang of the link between muscle tension and mental stress, you'll be better equipped to spot and fight off stress symptoms.

Diaphragmatic Breathing Exercises are your go-to for quickly **clearing** your mind, showcasing just how much controlled breathing can impact your anxiety levels. The "4-7-8" technique is a nifty little **trick** you can use every day to keep stress at arm's length.

Autogenic Training and self-suggestion are fantastic for diving into deep relaxation and achieving mental clarity. They're like a **reset** button for your mind.

By weaving these stress-busting techniques into your life, you're setting yourself up for improved mental well-being and a more **balanced** existence. Make them a regular part of your routine, and you'll see a real difference in how you handle stress and overthinking. Keep at it, stay **resilient**, and keep working on managing your stress effectively – it'll pay off big time!

Chapter 10: Building Mental Strength

Ever felt like your brain's doing a marathon and it's all uphill? We've all been there. But stick with me. This chapter? It's gonna make you **tough**. Yeah, you—you'll come away feeling **stronger**, sharper, ready to take on whatever life throws your way.

You see, building **mental** strength isn't just some goal—it's the key to facing **challenges** head-on. Imagine being able to handle tough situations without breaking a sweat. Easy? Maybe not. Possible? Absolutely.

Throw in some mad **problem-solving** tricks, and who wouldn't want a mind like that? You'll learn ways to make quicker, smarter **choices** and stand tall with newfound **confidence**. Plus, there's a whole how-to section for flexing those mental muscles.

I promise, by the end, you're gonna be so ready to **crush** whatever obstacles loom ahead. Dive in and let's toughen up that noggin!

Developing Mental Toughness

Ever been caught in an endless loop of bad thoughts? It's like being stuck in quicksand. The more you **struggle**, the deeper you sink. This is where mental toughness comes in—it's your rope to pull you out. By building mental strength, you're less likely to get trapped in a web of overthinking and pessimism. You start to have a **resilient** mind that brushes off the negatives.

Mental toughness, at its core, means you can handle life's challenges without crumbling. Think of it as your brain muscle. Just as you lift weights to grow stronger physically, you can train this muscle too. It consists of a few key parts: **confidence**, focus, and emotional control.

Confidence, the first component, instills a belief in your abilities. When you believe in yourself, you're less likely to doubt every decision or be afraid of outcomes. This reduces the number of times you fall into that nasty quicksand of overthinking. Imagine facing a tough situation with full certainty. You wouldn't waste time second-guessing—maybe you'd even tackle it head-on.

Focus is another piece. Ever tried to get something done but found your mind wandering to everything that might go wrong? Focus keeps your mind on what needs doing right now, not on potential missteps. It's like having a spotlight in a dark room, guiding you to the exits without stumbling over stuff. With better focus, you steer clear of useless worries.

Emotional control ties it all together. Life throws curveballs, and emotions can run wild. But if you can manage those **emotions**, you don't act purely on impulse or let minor setbacks ruin your day. You become like a rock in a storm—steady and calm. Think of kids handling school exams. The ones who control their nerves often do better, 'cause they're not lost in panic.

Each of these components helps you bounce back from curveballs life throws. With confidence, you handle insults or failures way better. Focus ensures you get back on track, even if you're thrown a bit off-course. Emotional control helps you pick yourself up without an emotional rollercoaster.

But how do you build mental toughness? One useful technique is the "**adversity** quotient." It measures how you respond to difficult situations. Instead of crumbling under stress, this method lets you see setbacks as challenges you can learn from. Imagine life as a series of mountains; some days, you're on top, and others, you're climbing. The adversity quotient tells you how well you cope.

First, you assess your current level of resilience—how do you typically handle bad days or disappointments? From there, you tackle everyday problems bit by bit, instead of avoiding them. Start with smaller issues, build confidence, and gradually face bigger ones. Over time, you'll find yourself stronger and less likely to drown in overthinking.

So, think about your last setback. Did it feel like the end of the world? That might've been because your mental resilience wasn't as high. By boosting your adversity quotient, you train your brain to look at challenges differently. Instead of seeing them as dead-ends, you view them as forks in the road, offering new paths.

There you have it! Building mental **toughness** isn't a walk in the park, but it's doable. With more confidence, focus, and emotional control, plus a higher adversity quotient, you're better equipped to resist falling into the overthinking trap. You bounce back faster and rise stronger. Here's to toughening up that brain muscle and winning more of those mental **battles**!

Improving Problem-Solving Skills

To tame the **overthinking** beast, good problem-solving skills are a must. Why? Well, when you handle stuff better, your mind starts to calm down. That big ball of anxiety? It gets smaller because you know how to tackle issues head-on instead of letting them swirl around in your head. You've probably noticed that when you solve a problem efficiently, there's this sudden lightness. Almost like a weight lifted off your shoulders. Our brains love clarity and hate chaos.

So, how do you harness the power of organized **problem-solving**? It's pretty simple. Imagine your problem is like a tangled ball of yarn. You just need a step-by-step plan to untangle it. Start by defining what's the actual issue. Sometimes what looks like a problem is just a symptom of something else. Knowing this makes the problem less overwhelming.

Next up, gather whatever info you need. Ask around, do a little research, whatever it takes. Don't try to fly blind. It's like assembling pieces of a jigsaw puzzle. Once you've got all the pieces in front of you, start **brainstorming** solutions. Go wild at this stage, don't censor yourself. Once you've got your list, weigh the pros and cons of each. There's no rush, take your time and assess which option feels best. Finally, just choose one and execute it. See if it works, and if it doesn't, tweak it until it does.

Speaking of methods, ever heard of the IDEAL **strategy**? It's a neat framework for sorting out even the trickiest dilemmas. IDEAL stands for Identify, Define, Explore, Act, and Look back. Let's break it down:

• Identify the Problem: Yeah, just get to the heart of what's bugging you. Sounds basic, but sometimes you're so tangled in stress that you don't see the root cause.

• Define Goals: Know what your endgame is. What's the best outcome you're shooting for? This way, you can keep your eyes on the prize and not get lost in side issues.

• Explore Possible Solutions: This stage is all about **creativity**. List down any and all solutions that come to mind. Nothing's too silly or too out there at this point. You might surprise yourself with an unexpectedly brilliant idea.

• Act on the Decision: Pick the most viable option and go with it. Don't procrastinate. Action deflates overthinking.

• Look Back: This is like a debrief. How did it go? What worked, what didn't? Learning from your process is gold. It makes you way better prepared for next time.

Shifting from **anxiety** to action is more than just calming. It's empowering. All these steps make the fogginess in your mind clear up, and that endless loop of worry slows down. Over time, you get quicker and better at it.

So, there you have it. Good problem-solving doesn't just manage issues; it transforms your whole approach to **stress**. Your mind thrives on patterns and **strategies** that work. You've got all you need, just try putting it into practice.

Enhancing Decision-Making Abilities

Ever get stuck trying to make a choice? You know, when you just can't seem to **decide** and end up overthinking everything? That's called analysis paralysis. When you boost your **confidence** in making decisions, you can really cut back on those endless cycles of worrying. Fear of making the wrong choice can be a real killer. But when you're sure of yourself, that fear starts to disappear.

When you make a confident decision, you don't have to mull over every little detail forever. Sure, there will always be things you can't control. But making a **choice** and sticking with it can save you so much mental energy. And guess what? Mental energy matters. It means you're not wasting brainpower on stuff that doesn't really need it. That energy can then go to more important things.

So how can being decisive lower your **stress** levels? Good question. It's like this: when you're not stressing over multiple options, your mind is clearer. You've picked a path and you're walking it. This clarity means you've got less mess floating around in your head.

Instead of juggling ten different possibilities, you're on solid ground. That's going to create a calmer state of mind.

Ever noticed how a cluttered room makes you feel chaotic? Making a decision can be like cleaning up that room. You toss out what's unnecessary and keep only what matters. It's really freeing. And trust me, there's a lot of peace of mind when you're decisive. It gives you **purpose**, direction. You're not walking through life aimlessly, wondering if you made the right call on every tiny thing.

So how do you make a good decision without second-guessing yourself? There's a cool method called "pros and cons analysis." Okay, hear me out. Grab a piece of paper or just think about it in your head. Write down or visualize the **benefits** and drawbacks of each option. Keep it simple.

Imagine you're trying to figure out if you should move to a new city for a job. On one side, you list the good stuff: better salary, new adventure, chance to grow. On the other side, the not-so-good stuff: leaving friends behind, cost of living, uncertainty.

Seeing everything laid out can help you weigh things properly. No super computer needed. When you boil it down, it helps you see the choice more clearly. It's not this huge, intimidating decision anymore. It's just a bunch of points, some good, some bad. And once you've weighed it all, making the choice isn't as scary.

Alright, so to wrap this up... yes, being more confident and **decisive** goes a long way to beat overthinking. The clearer mind that comes with decisiveness can't be overstated. Clearing out that mental clutter reduces stress and makes you feel way better. Shut down doubts with a good pros and cons list. And get on with living instead of second-guessing.

Incorporate these tools and watch how your decisions get faster, simpler, and less stressful. Trust me, you'll find that life feels a whole lot less like a guessing game and more like you're in control. Decisiveness is like a muscle. The more you use it, the stronger it gets. So, in the end, making **decisions** will feel as easy and straightforward as chatting with an old friend.

Boosting Self-Confidence

You've probably heard it a thousand times: **confidence** is key. But you might be wondering, key to what exactly? Well, it's kind of like armor for your mind. When you boost your self-confidence, you create a shield against self-doubt and overthinking. Imagine every time you're second-guessing yourself, that confidence shield lights up and shoves those bad thoughts away. Pretty cool when you think about it, right?

Let me tell you about my friend Sarah. She always used to **overthink** and worry about her decisions, big or small. She'd stew over an email for hours. But quietly, she started working on her self-confidence. Little by little, she noticed that self-doubt popping up less and less. Gradually, she started making decisions quickly. No more sleepless nights wondering if she had ruined everything with a single click of "send".

So, why does this work? Well, when you genuinely **believe** in your abilities, there's less room, or even need, for worry. When you're confident, you're less likely to trouble yourself with "what ifs." Basically, less fretting means less **anxiety**. You walk around feeling sure and certain. Pretty calm, right?

Imagine riding a bike. When you're learning, you're wobbly and anxious about falling. But when you get the hang of it—smooth sailing. Same thing with confidence in your abilities. You simply stop worrying about every bump in the road. And honestly, it's incredible how powerful this belief can be.

Now, imagine you want to capture this confidence and build on it. Enter the "**confidence log**." Think of it as your personal cheerleader, the journal that helps you see your wins. Anytime you do something you're proud of, scribble it down. A tricky work task you nailed, motivating yourself to hit the gym, or perhaps that killer presentation at work—you name it.

Writing in the confidence log means that, when doubt comes knocking, you whip out the journal. Reading your **achievements** helps remind you of what you're capable of. It's so easy to forget your wins when you're focusing on the bumps along the way. Basically, you're making a record of proof. Proof that you've been beating these hurdles one by one.

Here's how you can start:

• Get yourself a journal. Doesn't have to be anything fancy.

• Set a time each day or week to jot down your achievements. Big or small.

• Include how these moments made you feel.

Keeping this log isn't just helpful for immediate boosts. It builds a library of evidence that you're pretty awesome. Over time you'll start to see patterns. Maybe you notice you're good at problem-solving. Or you might find out you're becoming a better team player. It all adds up to higher self-confidence.

And with this growing self-assurance, you start handling life's stuff with ease. Little problems stay little. You aren't giving in to those nagging thoughts anymore. It's like flexing a **muscle**. The more you use it, the stronger it gets. And with all that strength, overthinking doesn't stand a chance.

So, ready to lock out self-doubt and overthinking? Start building that confidence right away. Thought by thought, log by log.

This chapter certainly isn't going to miraculously change everything in an instant, but slowly, you'll find yourself looking back and wondering why you wasted so much time doubting yourself. You're becoming a stronger version of you—one **confident** decision at a time.

Practical Exercise: Mental Strength Training Plan

Let's dive into how you can **train** your mind to be stronger. First up, think of three tough situations you often face. It could be anything that **stresses** you out or makes you uncomfortable. Your daily grind, arguments, or big decisions at work. Jot 'em down.

Those tough spots? They're your mental **growth** playground. They're where it all starts.

Now that you've pinpointed some tricky situations, it's time to talk yourself up. For each one, come up with a positive self-talk **statement**. Might sound cheesy, but trust me, it works. Something like, "I've got this," or "I've handled worse before."

Positive self-talk is your secret weapon against those stormy mental days. It's like a ray of sunshine giving you an instant **boost**.

Ever tried tackling problems with a game plan? Here's a nifty method: the IDEAL approach. Pick one tough situation and work through these steps:

• Identify the problem

• Define the best outcome

• Explore all possible solutions

• Act on the best option

• Look back to evaluate success

Think of it like fixing a bike. Step-by-step, you handle each part until everything's running smoothly. So take that tough situation and give the IDEAL method a whirl.

With problem-solving in motion, let's switch gears. **Decisions** can be mind-boggling, right? Whip up a quick pros and cons list for a choice you need to make. List the good and the bad side-by-side.

Pros and cons sharpen your personal analysis, making decisions less of a headache.

Next up, let's bask in some positivity. Focus on your personal **strengths** or achievements. Write down three in your confidence log. This isn't about bragging; it's about reminding yourself what you bring to the table.

Writing boosts your self-esteem. It's like a quick mood pick-me-up.

Now, let's talk **goals**. Set one small, totally doable goal for the next week. Maybe finish that book you started or go for a run. Small goals push you bit by bit, like planting seeds in a garden.

Setting goals means chasing progress, not perfection.

Finally, it's time to mull it all over. Reflect on how each exercise affects your tendency to **overthink**. How did self-talk change your mindset? Did pros and cons simplify choices? Scribble down your thoughts.

Reflection reveals your mental habits. It's closing the loop.

Keeping things breezy and actionable cuts down on that mental clutter. Life doesn't have to feel like you're constantly navigating a maze. With each step, your mental strength grows. Like watering a plant, your soul gets lighter, your mind clearer, and life breezier.

Conclusion

Building mental strength is crucial for fighting off overthinking and negative thoughts. This chapter dives into several techniques and methods that are key to developing mental resilience. By putting these strategies into action, you can level up your **problem-solving skills**, sharpen your decision-making, and give your self-confidence a real boost.

Here's what you should take away:

• Mental toughness is your shield against overthinking and negative thoughts.

• The core components of mental toughness play a huge role in how resilient you are.

• The adversity quotient technique helps you build mental resilience by flipping challenges into opportunities.

• Systematic problem-solving is your ticket to less anxiety and a clearer mind.

• Confident decision-making can seriously cut down on stress and mental clutter.

As you get to grips with these ideas, you'll be **better equipped** to face life's curveballs with a positive attitude. So, make sure you put what you've learned in this chapter into practice in your day-to-day life. You'll see your mental resilience and confidence grow stronger with each passing day. You'll become a pro at **tackling challenges**, solving problems like a boss, and making decisions with more confidence than ever. Keep pushing forward, and unlock your full potential!

I'm excited for you to see how these **strategies transform** your life. Remember, it's all about consistent practice and patience. You've got this!

Chapter 11: Creating Healthy Habits

Ever wonder why you can't stick to those **goals** you set every New Year? Well, I've been there too. This chapter might be the **key** you need. Imagine waking up every day refreshed, eating **food** that powers your brain, feeling great after moving your body, and actually achieving the goals you set. Yeah, it sounds awesome, right?

As you dive into this chapter, you'll start seeing how little **changes** can make a big impact. We're talking improving how you **sleep**, what you eat, how you **exercise**, and setting goals that you'll actually meet. And it's all doable. Pretty soon, those **habits** will start clicking into place. I really believe in what I'm sharing here. Ready to shake things up and see the difference? You won't believe how simple changes can transform your **life**. Trust me—by the end of this chapter, you'll be eager to get moving.

Establishing a Consistent Sleep Routine

Getting good sleep is one of the best ways to stop **overthinking**. When your mind's well-rested, everything seems clearer. You're not fighting through a fog. Your thoughts feel easier to handle, even when things get stressful. Have you noticed? After a solid night of sleep, solutions come quicker. Overthinking? Not so much.

Think about how a lack of sleep affects you. Ever had one of those nights where you just can't drift off? Your mind is running in circles, going over every little thing. Next day? You're grumpy, decisions take forever, and everything feels out of control. Consistent sleep digs you out of that hole. It's like giving your **brain** a good clean-up every night.

Your brain's kinda like a car engine. After running all day, it needs downtime to cool off and get ready for another drive. While you sleep, your brain's working. It processes info, repairs itself, and sorts out **emotions**. When we talk sleep, we also talk feelings. Without enough shut-eye, feelings get out of whack. Little things become a big deal. Mood swings? Totally a thing.

So, how do you get better sleep? There's something called "sleep **hygiene**." It's not about showers before bed, though that could help. We're talking habits. Here's a quick checklist to get your routine down:

• Same Time Every Night - Consistency is king. Try to hit the hay at the same hour daily. Your body's clock will thank you.

• No Screens Before Bed - Those screens do a number on your melatonin. Try ditching them an hour before sleep. Read a book or listen to some calming music instead.

• Make Your Bedroom a Sanctuary - Keep it cool, quiet, and dark. Invest in comfortable bedding. Your sleep space should invite rest.

• Mind Your Munchies - Big meals, caffeine, and booze close to bedtime are bad news. They mess with your sleep rhythm. Keep it light in the evenings.

• Exercise, but Not Late - Physical activity is great, but hitting the gym late can keep you wired. Aim for earlier in the day.

With these tips on board, quality sleep becomes a reality, not a dream.

Alright, moving from good habits to how sleep shapes your brain and moods. Think of sleep as your brain's refresh button. Without it, cognitive **functions** like memory and decision-making go south. Your alertness? Almost non-existent. We talked emotions—picture your brain drowning without enough sleep. You can't cope as well. Challenges turn into crises. You get snappier, less patient.

Healthy sleep habits can help you master emotions and cut down **stress**. Think of it like building a strong foundation for sanity. No more unnecessary drama piling up.

Finally, let's talk about why these habits are tools for keeping overthinking at bay. Ever tried solving puzzles when you're tired? Frustrating, right? Imagine setting lifelong puzzles for yourself. Sleep declutters your mind, shifts out the junk, makes way for clear thoughts. Keeps that mind treadmill from spinning into overdrive.

You, armed with good sleep, are the master of your mind's game. Create a habit following this checklist, and see how your **perspective** changes. Like flipping a switch, habits for restful sleep tune up your mental gear. From less overthinking, improved moods, to sharper mind functions—your ticket to a calmer existence starts at bedtime.

Nutrition for Mental Clarity

Let's get straight into it. **Eating** right isn't just about fitting into your favorite jeans. It's your **brain's** best friend. When you fuel your body with good food, your brain stays sharp, focused, and less anxious. Think of the mind as a machine that runs on the fuel you give it.

Ever noticed you feel groggy or anxious after munching on junk? That's no accident. The relationship between what you eat and how you think is significant. Load yourself with junk food, and you'll notice your brain getting sluggish and overrun with anxious thoughts. On the flip side, feeding yourself nutritious food equates to a clear mind and a decrease in everyday worries.

Next up, **gut** health. Bet you didn't think your stomach was calling the shots up there in your brain. But it is. The gut-brain axis is a real thing, and your digestion is linked to your mood. Gut-friendly foods keep your stomach calm and show your mind some love.

Think about it like this: a healthy gut means happier thoughts. Ever heard of serotonin? It's often called the "happy chemical," and a whopping 90% of it is produced in your gut. So, keeping your belly content with good bacteria leads to a happier mind. Yogurt, leafy greens, and fibrous veggies are your go-tos here. Keep your gut flora happy, and they'll return the favor by lifting your spirits.

Now, let's visualize the **foods** making the magic happen. Here's where the "brain-boosting meal plan" shines. It's about eating the right blend that keeps your mind sharp and mood bright. This isn't about strict diets or cutting everything you love—it's tweaking what you eat to help your brain run smoother.

Breakfast should be simple but powerful. Start your day with whole grains, protein, and fruits. Think oatmeal with a sprinkle of nuts and fresh berries. Maybe a slice of whole-grain toast with avocado. These options offer steady energy, reducing the peaks and valleys that can lead to tiredness and despair.

For **lunch**, mix in some lean proteins and plenty of greens. A grilled chicken salad loaded with colorful veggies can work wonders. Tofu or beans are great for the plant-based crowd. Add a splash of olive oil to get your healthy fats in, and your brain will thank you.

Dinner should be about balance. Get your lean protein, more veggies, and some smart carbs like quinoa or brown rice. Omega-3 fatty acids are especially brain-friendly. Think salmon or walnuts. These support brain function and reduce anxiety.

Snacks between meals? Go nuts, but literally. Nuts, seeds, and a bit of dark chocolate can curb your hunger and sprinkle in some extra nutrients. They boost your concentration and keep that brain fog away.

So, what's the take-away? Eating right significantly betters your mental clarity, curbs anxious thoughts, and connects deeply with your gut health. It's not just about feeding your body but nurturing your mind. Make small, smart changes to your diet, and notice the way it changes your mind. Happy munching!

Regular Exercise for Mental Health

You can't deny that **exercise** makes you feel good. When you're stressed out, working out is like hitting a reset button. Your worrying starts to dial back, and suddenly things don't look so bad. Picture this: you're on a treadmill or going for a jog, and instead of thinking about whatever's bugging you, you're focusing on your steps, your breathing, the rhythm. It's almost magical how physical movement flips off that anxiety switch in your head.

Working out doesn't just cut down stress. It perks up your whole mood. You know when you eat chocolate and get that rush of happiness? That's because your brain is getting a hit of feel-good chemicals. Exercise has a similar effect, but without the sugar crash. Just twenty or thirty minutes of moving your body gets those endorphins flowing and serotonin levels rising. Suddenly, you're not just okay—you're on top of the world. And this isn't the kind of high that fizzles out quickly. This **mood boost** sticks around, like a happy afterglow that carries you through the day.

Now, let's talk about what happens in your **brain** when you exercise. Imagine all those brain fog moments and negative thoughts draining away like water through a sieve. When you stick to a routine, your memory gets sharper, you can focus more easily, and you even tend to sleep better. It's like your brain's cleaning crew comes through, tidying up and making things run smoothly again.

Your brain gets a literal workout during physical activity. Blood flow increases, taking more oxygen and nutrients with it. It's as if your brain's been given a turbo boost, helping it function at its best. So, if you're feeling cloudy or bogged down by overthinking, grab those sneakers and get moving. You'll feel clearer, sharper, and—dare I say it—happier.

With all that great stuff going on, wouldn't it be nice to have a go-to routine to rely on? Enter the "**mood-boosting workout** routine." Think of it as a handy toolbox. This one's tailored to keep stress and anxiety at bay. You don't need a gym membership. Just some space and a little willpower.

Here's a simple plan:

• Warm-Up: Start with 5 minutes of stretching or light jogging on the spot.

• Cardio Burst: 15 minutes of jumping jacks, running, or dancing to your favorite tunes. Anything that gets your heart pumping.

• Strength Training: 10 minutes of bodyweight exercises like push-ups, squats, or lunges. Mix it up so you don't get bored.

• Cool Down: Spend the last 5 minutes stretching and doing breathing exercises.

After just one session, you might feel like you've pushed a mental refresh button. Over time, this routine helps keep **anxiety** and bad thoughts at bay. Your brain and body thank you for it.

Exercise really is a game-changer for **mental health**. From cutting down stress to improving brain function and offering a handy routine to support your mood, it ticks all the boxes. Give it a go and see how much better you feel.

Setting SMART Goals

Overthinking often happens when you don't know what you want or where you're headed. Setting clear **goals** can act like a roadmap. It helps you cut through all the pointless thoughts that can crowd your mind. Goals give you **direction**—like turns and stops on a trip. So instead of wandering about, wondering what to do next, you've got a plan. It's much easier to focus on what matters when you're not bogged down by unnecessary worries.

There's something called SMART goals. They sound technical but really, they're just about making your goals clearer. SMART stands for Specific, Measurable, Achievable, Relevant, and Time-bound. Let's break them down:

• Specific: Instead of saying "get fit," say "run three times a week."

• Measurable: Something you can track. "Lose 10 pounds" rather than just "lose weight."

• Achievable: It has to be something you can actually do. Don't aim to run a marathon in a month if you've never run before.

• Relevant: It should mean something to you. A goal like "learn to cook" makes more sense if you enjoy cooking or eating well.

• Time-bound: Give yourself a deadline. "Read 12 books this year" is clearer than just "read more."

Setting up goals like this helps you **grow** because it's like building a staircase instead of climbing a sheer cliff—you move up step-by-step. That makes personal **growth** more manageable. When you define things clearly, you understand what you need to do next. This lessens the chances of getting lost in a sea of thoughts.

So, how do you actually make these SMART goals work for you? Start small. Identify one area of your life where you feel like you're overthinking or not making progress. Maybe it's your health, your job, or even a hobby. Pick one thing to focus on. For instance, if it's your health, you might decide to "walk 30 minutes every day for a month."

Write it down—really, it helps. Seeing your goal on paper makes it tangible. Note all the aspects: "You will walk (specific) 30 minutes (measurable) each day (achievable) because you want to be healthier (relevant), for the next 30 days (time-bound)."

Next, figure out how you're going to measure your **progress**. It could be a checkmark on a calendar or a note on your phone. Tracking this way gives you a sense of accomplishment every time you complete a step—you'll know you're moving forward.

Adjust as you go. Life's unpredictable, and sometimes things don't go as planned. If you miss a couple of walks, don't beat yourself up. Just adjust your goal if needed and keep moving forward. **Flexibility** is key here—you're not chiseling these goals in stone. You're writing them down to have a direction.

And once you achieve a SMART goal? Celebrate. Reward yourself for sticking to it. Successful goal-setting builds **momentum**. Every step you take, no matter how small, makes the next one easier. Slowly but surely, you'll find yourself spending less time in your head and more time living your life as you wish.

And that's what SMART goals are all about. Taking charge, setting a clear direction, and moving forward, step-by-step. It sounds simple because, at its core, it really is. The power lies in clarity and focus. No more wandering aimlessly or second-guessing yourself. You know where you're headed, and you have a plan to get there.

In Conclusion

This chapter offers **simple** tips and tricks for creating **healthy** habits that can boost your mental well-being, help control **overthinking**, and reduce **stress**. The main focus areas include sleep, nutrition, **exercise**, and goal-setting. By tweaking your daily **routine**, you can set yourself up for a happier and healthier mind.

You've learned that quality **sleep** is crucial for reducing overthinking and improving mental clarity. Eating the right foods can really help your brain function better and lift your mood. Regular exercise not only keeps your body in shape but also gives your spirits a boost. **SMART** goals can help you stay on track and avoid unnecessary worry. Following step-by-step guides can make it easier to form and stick to these healthy habits.

So why not give these simple steps a try? Add them to your routine, and you'll start to notice a big change in your mood and thought patterns. The steps are easy to follow, and they can really help you lead a more relaxed and focused life. Go for it!

Chapter 12: Positive Psychology in Action

Ever wonder why some days just feel **better** than others? You've been there. You, too, could experience that steady good vibe if you knew what to look for. This chapter will guide you through some pretty neat ways to **spice** up your day-to-day life.

Have you thought about how practicing **gratitude** might flavor your outlook? When you start paying more attention to the little things, it's a game-changer. You can try it, too. Savoring those positive **experiences**? It's so, so worth it. It'll change the way you see everything, trust me.

Want more? I bet you do. Picture immersing yourself in **activities** that make you forget time exists. That's engaging in flow activities — something unbelievably satisfying. Then, there's the magic of keeping a sunny **outlook**. Even when things get tough, holding on to optimism opens up new possibilities.

And before we wrap things up, there's a practical **exercise** for you— the Positivity Boost Toolkit. It's packed with stuff you can start using right away. Ready to see your days light up? Dig in and feel the **change** yourself—it'll be worth it.

Practicing Gratitude

Ever notice how easy it is to fall into a negative thought spiral? It's like once you start thinking negatively, everything seems worse.

Stuff you never even thought about before just pops up, making you feel even more down. This is where practicing **gratitude** comes in. By focusing on the good things, you can shift your whole **outlook**. Instead of constantly thinking about what's going wrong, you'll start noticing what's going right. Imagine that!

Picture coming home after a rough day at work. Your boss was on your case, traffic was awful, and it feels like nothing's going your way. But then you start to think about the little things – a coworker brought you coffee, a car let you merge into traffic, or the sunset was particularly beautiful. Such thoughts can seriously make a **difference**.

Or, think about how appreciating the roof over your head or the food on your table can change your **mood**. These thoughts don't have to be profound or life-changing. Just the simple things that we often take for granted. Practicing gratitude forces your brain to switch gears, and over time, you start seeing your life through a more positive lens.

Speaking of the brain, let's talk about what gratitude does up there. When you're genuinely thankful, your brain experiences a kind of workout, releasing feel-good chemicals like serotonin and dopamine. They're like the body's natural mood lifters. Pretty cool, right? Gratitude shifts your mindset from "what's broken" to "what's working." This shift not only lifts your spirits but lowers **stress**. Your whole body responds like a big sigh of relief.

Stress doesn't stand a chance against a grateful heart. Imagine you're hustling day in and day out, surrounded by stressors – bills, deadlines, responsibilities – but for a few moments each day, you pause to just think about the good stuff. This brings calm and perspective.

Now, let's get practical. You're probably wondering how to incorporate gratitude into your daily grind without it being another chore. This is where the "three good things" method steps in. Each night before you hit the hay, jot down three positives about your day. They don't have to be major **events**. Maybe your coffee was extra delicious or you got a warm message from a friend. This practice rewires your brain to notice these good moments instinctively.

Picture sitting down with a notebook and recalling three positive moments. It's not just for feel-good vibes; you're training your brain to see the upside, lessening the load of those stressful days.

It's amazing how **consistency** can transform your mindset. The more you practice, the more effortless gratitude becomes. Soon, you'll find yourself spotting the good in the middle of chaos – like finding tiny pockets of joy amid life's hustle. Even a rough day won't faze you as much because your brain will be like, "Hey, it's still a good life!"

So, make "three good things" a nightly **habit**. It's simple and takes just a few minutes. Over time, these small acts of gratitude can bring a wave of positivity, shifting your whole perspective on life. And you'll probably sleep better too. Cheers to a more grateful, less stressful life – it's easier than you think.

Savoring Positive Experiences

Ever find yourself lost in thoughts, **worrying** about the past or future? It's like your brain decides to throw a little party for every single anxious thought you've ever had. Not so fun, right? But there's a way out. **Enjoying** the moment — yep, that's the ticket. Taking time to really soak up the good stuff happening around you can actually make you feel better. Let's see how.

Think about something simple, like eating a piece of chocolate. If you just toss it in your mouth and chomp it down, did you really enjoy it? Probably not. But if you let it melt slowly, paying attention to the taste, the texture, the way it makes you feel... suddenly, it's like this little sensory adventure. This is what we mean by **savoring** the moment.

When you're caught up in enjoying these little experiences, there's less room for worrying. Instead of thinking about that awkward conversation you had yesterday or stressing about tomorrow's meetings, you're fully present. It's like giving your brain a mini-vacation. Focusing on the good stuff can send the bad thoughts packing. Sounds neat, huh?

Let's dive into how positive feelings are so helpful for your mind. Boosting those good vibes isn't just about feeling happy for a moment. It's deeper than that. When you tap into positive **emotions**, you're literally changing the way your brain works. Science backs this up.

Positive emotions can lower stress hormones. So, the more you smile, laugh, or enjoy life, the better your mental **health** gets. It's a bit like compounding interest in a savings account—the benefits keep adding up. It can improve how you deal with stress and even sharpen your mind! Less thinking, worrying... and more living.

Feeling good is like having a superhero in your back pocket. It helps you bounce back faster from setbacks. You're better at handling the daily grind. Who wouldn't want that kind of mental boost? So, to feel better and think less, piling up those good moments is a must.

Speaking of moments, let's wrap this up with a cool way to savor good experiences: the "savoring walk." Here's the deal. This isn't just any walk. You go outside, leave your worries behind, and tune into every little thing that pleases you. Simple concept but super effective.

As you walk, notice the details. Maybe it's how the sunlight filters through the leaves or the sound of birds chirping. Even the crunch of gravel under your feet can be delightful if you pay attention. What you're doing is focusing on nice **sensations**, one at a time. It keeps your mind too busy with positives to wander off into worry-land.

Here's a fun tip—try doing this with a buddy. You can both point out things you find enjoyable. It's a way of doubling the feel-good factor because you're sharing the joy. And who said feeling better had to be a solo trip anyway?

So, if **overthinking** ever becomes too much, take a walk. Notice the world around you. Enjoy each moment. Before you know it, your mind calms down, and you're no longer tangled in unwanted thoughts. You'll discover that savoring good experiences helps fight off overthinking and boosts **happiness**.

Engaging in Flow Activities

Ever get so lost in something that time just flies? That's what we call a **flow** state. It's one of the best ways to give your mind a break from overthinking. Just like when a good movie pulls you in and you forget about everything else.

Flow can be your natural **escape**. When you're deep into a flow activity, there's no room for stress or bad thoughts. Imagine jogging through your favorite park, painting, or even playing a complex video game—it's like flipping a switch. Your brain focuses completely on the task at hand. Suddenly, all those looping thoughts just disappear.

But how does this magic work? Well, let's think about the psychological stuff behind it. Flow isn't just a fancy term; it's got real **science** backing it. You feel balanced between your challenge and your skill level. If it's too easy, you get bored. Too hard, you get frustrated. But when it's just right, like a perfect match, you get engaged. Time either flies by or seems to stop. You're fully present, and it's basically like your brain is getting a mini-vacation.

Here's the cool part: flow makes you feel genuinely happier. Science says it reduces cortisol—yeah, that stress stuff. So, not only are you busy having fun, but you're also getting invisible mental perks along the way. It's a win-win.

Alright, let's connect this idea to making it practical. We know flow is good. But how do you find your flow **activity**? Think about what you already love doing. Maybe it's cooking or repairing that old bike in your garage. Maybe it's rehearsing a piece of music you adore or gardening.

Start by listing things you enjoy. Easy, right? Now, ask yourself: does time stop when you do this? That's a good clue. Pick a few activities that meet this and set aside **time** for them regularly. It could be as simple as dedicating thirty minutes to write in your journal or sketch something. Flow doesn't have to be some rare thing; you can seamlessly include it in your life.

Once you've got your activities narrowed down, the next step is making them flow-friendlier. That's a word now—I just invented it! Structure and **challenge** are equally key. If you're into knitting, try a complex pattern versus something too simple. If it's jogging, maybe push your distance a bit gradually. Pushing your limits just enough keeps you engaged and right in that flow sweet spot.

Let's wrap this up. Flow activities aren't just about having fun. They're your gateway to stopping all that **overthinking**! Remember those times when your worries faded away while you were totally absorbed in something?

There are endless flow options out there. Crafting a little more flow in your daily **routine** isn't tough. Grab a paintbrush, lace up those running shoes, strum that guitar. Soon enough, overthinking will be a thing of the past, and you'll be on a natural high.

Fostering Optimism

You know, it's **tricky** to stay upbeat when negative thoughts are rushing through your mind. But, realistic optimism comes to the rescue here. It helps you fend off those bad spirals that lead straight to anxiety city. This isn't about putting on rose-colored glasses; it's about seeing the good in situations while also recognizing the bad. For instance, you might have had a terrible day at work. Realistic optimism lets you say, "Yeah, today was rough, but I've handled such days before, and tomorrow's another chance." You're not ignoring the struggle—you're just choosing to not be swallowed by it.

When you focus on the positive possibilities amidst problems, you're retraining your **brain**. It's like planting seeds in your mind's garden. When you water these seeds with positive thoughts, you give less room for weeds of worry and fear to grow. It doesn't mean you'll never have a bad thought again, but with practice, you'll find it easier to redirect your mind to brighter avenues.

There's a big difference between blind optimism and learned **optimism**. Blind optimism is like walking into a storm thinking you won't get wet. It's neither realistic nor helpful. It ignores all signs of trouble and banks everything on pure wishful thinking, which can leave you feeling worse when things don't pan out.

On the flip side, learned optimism is grounded. It's taught. You gain it by practicing positive self-talk and recognizing the **control** you have over your reactions to events. You're not just hoping for the best—you're actively working towards it. Start small. Catch yourself when you're spiraling. Replace "I can't handle this" with "I've managed tough stuff before, and I can do it again."

Now, what can supercharge your optimistic outlook? It's a little technique called the "best possible self." Think about this: You sit down, close your eyes, and imagine yourself in the **future**. Not just any future, but the best one you can dream of. Picture all those things you want to achieve and the person you want to be. You see yourself happy, successful, and fulfilling your goals.

Doing this regularly primes your brain for optimism. It's like programming your mind to recognize the good stuff that's yet to come. Spend a few minutes every day visualizing this best version of yourself. Write it down if that helps you keep the vision clear. As you do this, you might feel a shift in your daily **mood**. You start to look at current challenges as steps leading you to this wonderfully optimistic future you've visualized.

But it's not all magic. This technique, while effective, needs a sprinkle of **persistence** and a dash of routine. The benefits build up over time. You might start noticing that things just don't weigh you down as much anymore. They're just little bumps on your road to becoming your 'best possible self'.

So, there you have it. Realistic optimism, distinct from blind faith, gives you true ground to stand on. Learned optimism is about building a muscle. And the "best possible self" is your daily **practice** for long-term positivity. Sounds doable, right?

Practical Exercise: Positivity Boost Toolkit

Feeling tangled in your own thoughts can be like trying to find your way out of a dense forest. It's easy to get lost. But with simple steps, you can clear those mental bushes. So let's start with **gratitude**.

Jot down three things you're thankful for today. It's amazing how something as simple as this can shift your **perspective**. Whether it's that first sip of morning coffee, a warm hug from a friend, or even just a sunny day, noting them down matters. You start to see the good around you, making it tougher for those pesky thoughts to take over.

Next, take a moment to think about a recent good **experience**. Got it? Excellent. Now, spend two minutes really appreciating it. Close your eyes if it helps and relive that moment. Smell the smells, hear the sounds, feel the feels. This trick works wonders 'cause it teaches your mind to focus on the bright spots, reminding you that it's not all doom and gloom out there.

Alright, now let's shift gears. Time to list three of your personal **strengths**. This one's sometimes tough. But trust me, you've got strengths. Are you kind? Brave? Good listener? Write 'em down! And think about how you've used these strengths recently. Maybe you offered support to a friend in need or solved a tricky problem at work. Acknowledging these makes you realize your own awesomeness and how you contribute to life around you.

Sliding into the next exercise—isn't it nice to plan something that fits with your values? Set a small, doable **goal** for the day. Nothing too flashy. It could be something like making your bed, giving someone a compliment, or spending a few minutes on a hobby. When your goals align with what you believe in, it gives you a boost without feeling like another chore.

Now, let's hit pause. Do a 5-minute loving-kindness **meditation**. Sit comfortably, close your eyes, and imagine sending love and goodwill towards yourself, then extend it outward to others. Yeah, meditating might sound fancy, but it's really just a moment of calm in the middle of chaos. You'll feel the tension slipping away bit by bit.

Ready to mix things up? Dive into an **activity** you enjoy for at least 15 minutes. Whether it's reading a book, taking a walk, or even doodling, just lose yourself in something fun. It gives your mind a break and brings a splash of joy to the day.

Finally, reflect on how these exercises affect your mood and thoughts. Feel any lighter? More grounded? More in control? Jot down your feelings. Doing these exercises can turn your day around, cutting through stress and letting you breathe easier. Over time, you'll notice some positive changes in how you think and feel. Isn't that the **goal**?

So, there you have it. Go through these steps like you're chatting with a friend over coffee. They're simple, but powerful. Keep at it, stay curious, and let these small actions become your positivity toolkit.

In Conclusion

This chapter has given you some **valuable** insights on how to use Positive Psychology in your everyday life. You've learned **powerful** techniques to boost your mental well-being. These strategies can help you feel **happier**, less stressed, and more optimistic. Here are the main points to keep in mind:

Gratitude can shift your focus from negatives to positives, making you feel better about life. Knowing how gratitude affects your **brain** can improve your mood and decrease stress. The "three good things" technique lets you jot down three things you're grateful for each day. **Savoring** positive experiences can increase your happiness and reduce overthinking. Understanding and practicing how **optimism** fights negative thoughts can lift your spirits.

Putting these ideas into practice will help you notice the **positive** aspects of life more easily. Give these techniques a whirl to see the benefits firsthand. Remember, each small effort makes a big difference! Keep practicing positive psychology, and watch how it **transforms** your outlook on life.

Chapter 13: Long-Term Strategies for Overthinking Prevention

Ever wonder why your **mind** runs a hundred miles a minute? I used to be just like you, wrestling with too many thoughts at all hours. Guess what? There's a way out. Think of this chapter as your **survival** kit for cutting off overthinking at the roots.

You're probably sick of feeling stuck and bogged down by your own **thoughts**. But in this chapter, you'll find some real game-changing stuff. I'll chat about building a killer **support** network and how setting **goals** that actually make sense will ease the mental overload. Along the way, you'll discover how to deal with **stress** like a pro and keep up with practices that constantly push you to **improve**. There's even a cool exercise to whip up your own plan for personal **growth**.

Let's dig in and get you on the track to a calmer, clearer head. You'll learn how to take control of your racing thoughts and find some much-needed peace. We'll explore practical strategies that'll help you nip overthinking in the bud and build a more balanced mindset.

From creating a rock-solid support system to setting achievable goals, you'll pick up tools that'll make a real difference in your day-to-day life. You'll also get the lowdown on stress management techniques that actually work, and discover how to keep yourself on a path of continuous improvement.

By the time you're done with this chapter, you'll have a tailor-made plan to tackle overthinking head-on. So, buckle up and get ready to transform your mental landscape. It's time to kiss those endless thought loops goodbye and hello to a more focused, relaxed you.

Building a Support Network

Feeling **bogged down** by overthinking? Spending time with friends and family could be your secret weapon to letting go of all that extra mental clutter. When you hang out with people who care about you, you get a break from all those nagging thoughts that won't leave you alone. Imagine hitting the reset button on your brain. Conversations, laughter, and just having someone to listen can change your entire outlook.

You don't have to talk about deep stuff all the time. Sometimes, simply watching a movie together or grabbing a cup of coffee can be enough. You see things from different angles when you're with others—angles that might never pop into your mind when you're all by yourself. Plus, you get to hear different opinions and stories, making your own worries seem a bit less gigantic. Just being around other people can **lighten** the emotional load you're carrying.

Let's be real, it's not just about getting new perspectives. Having someone to lean on when things get tough? That can seriously lower your **stress** levels. We all need a little help sometimes, and just knowing there's a buddy or family member willing to support you can make a world of difference. Stress isn't just in your head; it's in your whole body. When you're surrounded by support, you'll notice your shoulders might not feel so heavy anymore.

Leaning on others helps emotionally too. You learn that it's okay to feel what you're feeling, and that you don't have to go through it alone. Have you ever just talked something out and felt a lot better? It's like, out of nowhere, you realize things aren't as bad as you thought. Emotional relief is sometimes a simple phone call away. People who care will listen, and sometimes, that's all you need.

Moving on, let's talk about **maintaining** these essential bonds. Here's where the "relationship check-up" technique comes in handy. Yeah, it sounds a bit clinical, but it's super helpful. Think of it as taking the time here and there to evaluate your friendships and family relationships. Are they still strong? Are they still meaningful? This isn't just about figuring out who you should hang out with more or who maybe hasn't been as supportive as you'd like. It's about investing time in the relationships that truly matter.

When you notice a relationship could use a little nurturing, what do you do? Maybe it's time for an innocent catch-up over dinner. Or something as simple as a quick message to let them know you're thinking of them. Being proactive about your connections keeps them healthy, and strong relationships are less likely to contribute to your overthinking. Plus, these check-ups remind you of who really makes you feel good and who might be **draining**.

So chat with your parents, hang out with your buddies, or call an old friend. Letting your support network **buoy** you up can bring some serious — and much-needed — relief from the constraints of overthinking. After all, considering everything alone is exhausting. Recognizing that you have a community around you continually looking out for your well-being is **comforting**.

There you go! Some actionable steps for you to connect with the people around you. Build that support network because when times get rough, it's those relationships that will **pull** you through.

Setting Realistic Goals and Expectations

Setting goals is like a double-edged sword. If you're chasing perfection, it can lead to all kinds of anxiety and stress. But **balanced** goal-setting? That's a piece of magic for cutting down that perfectionist mindset.

Let's dive into balanced goal-setting. When you make goals that fit well with your current skills and resources, it pulls you away from the pesky habit of perfectionism. Picture this: setting a goal to stay **active** by walking outside for 20 minutes a day. It's easy to fit into your schedule, not overwhelming, and not some relentless gym routine. Perfect? No. Achievable? Absolutely. You'll start to see progress and feel good about it.

There's something special about hitting these manageable goals over and over. It gives you **confidence**, and that nasty need to be perfect starts to fade. Over time, balanced goals help you see results without drowning in endless self-criticism. Plus, your mind starts to relax because the targets you've set aren't out of this world. They're normal, doable, and keep you moving forward without the sky-high pressure.

Now, let's talk about the idea of "good enough." It's a simple yet potent way to knock down overthinking. Perfection is, let's be honest, not realistic. All it does is pull you into endless cycles of worry. Accepting something as "good enough" can be **liberating**. Say you're working on a project, and it's almost done but not flawless. A perfectionist would agonize over every little detail for hours, maybe even days. But aiming for good enough? You can finish things earlier, cut down on unnecessary stress, and still produce quality work.

This shift to "good enough" is crucial in how it cuts wasted time and worry. Imagine how much mental **energy** you save by not nitpicking everything. And remember, most of the time, your "good enough" is still pretty awesome. People will appreciate the effort you've put in, even if it's not absolutely perfect.

Let's move on to values-based goal setting—another clever trick. Here's the deal: when your goals flow from your core values, they mean more, and you're more likely to stay engaged. If family is a big part of your life, a goal like "dinner with family three times a week" isn't just another item on a checklist. It's something with personal **significance**, which keeps you on track and feeling connected.

By aligning your goals with your values, you're sticking close to what really matters. This way, you cut out a lot of unnecessary worry or dawdling. You're not just randomly setting goals to "achieve more." You're crafting them around what you care about, acting with **intention**, and not piling up stress.

All of these parts—balanced goals, accepting "good enough," and values-based goal setting—work together like gears in a reliable old watch. They keep things ticking along without the unnecessary jitters of striving for an impossible standard. Start each day grounding yourself in these practices, and watch as the overthinking starts to fall away. Instead of feeling burdened, you begin to navigate, reaching **milestones** easefully, one bit at a time. The journey becomes less about foolproof perfection and more about progress with purpose. So, here's to doing things well, enjoying the process, and reclaiming your calm mind.

Developing Coping Mechanisms

When you're facing **overthinking** triggers, having your own coping strategies can really help. I've leaned on several tried-and-true methods over the years, and let me tell you—having a go-to game plan makes a world of difference. It's all about finding what **works** for you. Maybe it's taking a walk, practicing some deep breathing, or chatting with a friend. Different strokes for different folks, right? Personally, I start my day with a bit of mindfulness. Just sitting quietly for five minutes sets the tone. Other times, it's all about **distraction**—cranking up some tunes or diving into a good book.

But not all coping ways are good for you. There's a big difference between ways that help and ways that hurt. Falling into bad habits, like smoking or hitting the bottle too hard, might seem like easy escapes. But in the long run, they only pile on more **stress**. It's like slapping a band-aid on a gaping wound. On the flip side, positive coping, like breaking a sweat or scribbling in a journal, actually tackles the root of the problem. For instance, when my thoughts start spiraling, I grab my **journal** and just let it all spill onto the page. It's like clearing out the mental clutter.

Linking these methods to a solid plan brings us to creating what I call a "coping **toolkit**." This toolkit is a collection of stress management tools you've tailor-made just for you. Think of it like a toolbox, but instead of wrenches and hammers, you've got breathing exercises, favorite playlists, and maybe some quick meditation apps. You don't need to fill it all at once. Build it up over time. Maybe start with the things you already know work, like that one song that always gets you grooving. And then, try out new stuff. Maybe yoga, or picking up a crafty hobby like knitting.

So, put together a small list. Here's how to do it. Jot down all the positive things that you know help you chill out or focus. Mix it up with a variety of activities. Some physical, like pounding the pavement or stretching. Some mental, like puzzles or reading. And some social, like ringing up a buddy or joining a group. Keep it somewhere easy to find. When overthinking creeps up, you'll have a ready-made set of tools to calm your mind. It's like having a shield against stress.

To wrap it all up, let's acknowledge that coping mechanisms take practice and **patience**. Sometimes, you'll try something, and it'll fall flat. That's okay. Chuck it out and try again. What's important is the effort you put into finding those little joys and tools that keep overthinking at bay. Think about the moments when you feel most at ease. If walking your dog brings peace, scribble that down. If doodling in a sketchbook makes a difference, add it to the list. It's all about knowing yourself and what makes your mind light up instead of shutting down.

So next time those stressful thoughts start bubbling up, you've got your toolkit ready to go. Little by little, you're going to find those overthinking episodes are fewer and farther between. Keep at it, and you'll be **mastering** your mind in no time.

Continuous Self-Improvement Practices

Let's chat about always striving to get **better**. You know, that desire to improve yourself bit by bit, day by day. It sounds simple, but it packs a punch. When you're constantly aiming to upgrade, it does something amazing for you—it makes you stronger against **overthinking**. Here's how.

By focusing on improvement, you keep your **mind** busy with stuff that's worth your time. You're thinking about opportunities, not dwelling on worst-case scenarios. So, if you're learning a new skill or habit, you don't have time to sit and stew over those endless "what ifs." You're moving forward, not getting stuck.

Always getting better also means you're tackling **challenges** head-on. You start small—maybe you decide to read one more chapter of a book each day. Over time, you're stacking up these small wins, which boosts your confidence. When you believe you can handle more, those mountains of worries start looking like mere molehills.

But how about your **brain** itself? It can actually change and help you think differently through a concept called neuroplasticity. Fancy term, but it basically means your brain's not set in stone. It can adapt and rewire itself based on your habits and experiences.

When you practice self-improvement, you're training your brain like a muscle. Pick up a new book or try mastering a new cooking recipe. What happens next is pure magic—your brain starts creating new connections. This helps in reshaping how you process thoughts, making it easier to steer clear of overthinking. So, more brain power on the good stuff, less on the habitual, bad thought patterns.

Now, let's switch gears. Say hello to something called the "**growth mindset challenge**." This is all about seeing learning opportunities everywhere. Whenever you face something tough, instead of thinking, "I can't do this," you flip the script. Challenges become just that—a chance to learn, rather than a chance to fail.

Here's how to put the growth mindset challenge to work for you. Start by picking something you've always wanted to learn. Maybe it's playing the guitar or speaking a new language. Next step? Dive into self-improvement through **practice**. But with a twist. You approach each stumble as a stepping stone. Made a mistake? Cool. That means you're learning.

This turns the tables on your usual anxious thoughts. Instead of fretting over mistakes or future failures, you're actively using each slip-up as a ladder rung. Over time, you're not just getting better at whatever you're doing; you're also getting better at managing your thoughts.

So, quick recap—keep bettering yourself to keep your mind from bad overthinking patterns. Your brain will actually reshape itself; give it something good to work with. And take on the growth mindset challenge to turn every hiccup into a learning moment.

These aren't isolated tricks. Imagine steering a boat. Constant self-improvement keeps your sails full of wind, propelling you forward. Neuroplasticity gives you a stronger, more adaptable boat. And the growth mindset challenge is like your trusty map, helping you see every gust of wind as a new direction to explore.

So, you see how each element plays into the other? It's a **system** that makes you stronger, more adaptable, and way better at dealing with those pesky overthinking moments. Keep these practices close, and you've got yourself a solid strategy for long-term prevention of overthinking.

Practical Exercise: Personal Growth Action Plan

Let's kick things off by figuring out which parts of your life you'd like to get better at. Think about your daily **routine**, your relationships, maybe even your hobbies. Pick three areas that you feel need some love and attention. Got them? Great, let's dig in.

Now you've got those three areas. Next up is setting some realistic, values-based **goals**. What does that mean, you ask? Values-based means something that's important to you, something that reflects what you care about. So, for each area, set one goal. Make sure it's achievable and stays true to what really matters to you. This could be anything like exercising more because health is important to you, or spending more time with family because they're a big part of your life.

So, you've got your goals. What next? Well, it's about making those goals less overwhelming. Break each one down into smaller, doable **steps**. For example, if your goal is exercising more, start with small actions like choosing three days a week for a 20-minute walk. Why? Because tiny steps are less daunting and a lot easier to tackle.

Alright, time to map out a plan. Take those smaller steps and make a **timeline** for the next month. Don't cram everything into a few days. Space things out to make the journey smoother. Let's use that exercise example. Maybe Week 1 is all about walking on Mondays, Wednesdays, and Fridays. By Weeks 2 and 3, you could aim for some light jogging mixed in. Watch how those small steps breathe life into your goal!

But what's a journey without a few stumbling blocks, right? Think about possible **roadblocks** and start planning ways to handle them. If bad weather could derail your walking routine, have a home workout ready. If a busy work week eats up family time, maybe schedule a family dinner over the weekend. That way, you're prepared when the universe throws you a curveball.

To stay on track, set up weekly **check-ins**. Look at how you're doing and make changes if needed. It's not about beating yourself up if you miss a step, it's about figuring out why you missed it and adjusting. Weekly check-ins can be short but super effective. Maybe jot down what went well and what could be better next time.

And hey, don't forget to celebrate little **wins**. These mini-successes add up and make the whole process fun. Like, if you managed all your workouts for Week 1, treat yourself to a movie night. If you nailed that family dinner, allow yourself some extra relaxation time. Plus, thinking about what you've learned along the way can give you valuable insights into yourself and your process.

There you have it: laying out your personal **growth** action plan. Start by picking the areas you care about, set realistic goals, break down the goals into steps, plan your timeline, think about possible hurdles, set up weekly check-ins, and celebrate along the way. It's a journey about growth and being kind to yourself through the process.

In Conclusion

This chapter has equipped you with some **valuable** tools and strategies to help keep your mind cool and stop yourself from overthinking. It's packed with great ideas to help you **build** better habits for the future. Let's quickly run through what you've learned.

Here's the lowdown on the key takeaways:

Your **friends** and family can be your secret weapon. Having solid social connections can help you see things more clearly and worry less. Plus, their support can be a real **stress-buster**, making you feel happier overall.

Don't forget about the "relationship inventory" technique. It's a nifty way to **figure** out which relationships in your life might need a little extra TLC.

When it comes to goals, think **smart**. Setting achievable targets helps you avoid stressing over everything being perfect. And here's a pro tip: when your goals align with your values, you end up achieving more **meaningful** things. It's like mind magic!

By putting these strategies into practice, you'll be well on your way to living a more **relaxed**, stress-free life. You'll be keeping that pesky overthinking at bay like a pro. Keep at it with what you've learned in this chapter, and I promise you'll see a **positive** change!

To Conclude

Ultimately, the true **goal** of this book has been to guide you out of the pitfalls of overthinking and toward a life filled with **clarity** and peace. You picked up this book because you were feeling overwhelmed by your thoughts and you sought effective ways to calm your mind, stop negative thinking, and relieve **stress**.

Let's shed light on what you've learned throughout these pages.

You now understand the weight that overthinking puts on your psychological well-being. You're equipped to recognize when you're stuck in this detrimental loop. You've learned that a positive shift in **mindset** can make a substantial difference.

You've got new tools to effectively reframe and manage your thoughts. You've got practical methods at your fingertips to interrupt your overthinking sessions instantly. Balancing out your thinking should now feel more achievable.

You've learned how to recognize, label, and express your **emotions** in a healthier way. You've honed your time-management skills to reduce the time available for overthinking. You've picked up valuable stress-reduction techniques that'll dampen your tendency to overthink.

You're reinforcing your capability to face **challenges** head-on and with confidence. You've learned about embedding healthy habits that can lead to sustained mental clarity. You've put positive psychology into action with tangible practices, making optimism more tangible in your life.

You've learned long-term strategies to continually stave off overthinking by building a support network, setting realistic goals, and continuously working on self-improvement.

Imagine a life where you're in control of your thoughts, and stress is no longer a chronic companion. By applying these tips and strategies, such a life is entirely within your reach. Each chapter you've worked through brings you one step closer to mental peace, **resilience**, and happiness.

To keep growing and expanding on what you've learned, keeping a support network and setting continuous developmental goals will pave the way for further transformation. Go forward with the confidence that you have the tools to keep overthinking at bay and foster a joyful, balanced life.

Visit this link to find out more:

https://pxl.to/LoganMind

Help Me!

When you support an independent author, you're supporting a **dream**.

When you're done reading and if you're satisfied, please consider leaving an honest **review**. Your **feedback** not only helps other readers discover the book but also aids in my growth as a writer.

If you've got suggestions for improvements, I'd be delighted to hear from you. Just shoot an email to the contacts you can find at the link below.

Alternatively, you can scan the QR code provided to easily access the review page.

Your review matters.

It only takes a few seconds, but your **voice** has a huge **impact**, encouraging and inspiring storytellers like myself to continue sharing our worlds and words with you.

Thanks for being a part of this **journey**.

Visit this link to leave feedback:

https://pxl.to/8-htson-lm-review

Join my Review Team!

Thank you for taking the time to read my **book**. Your support means the world to me. I'm excited to invite you to join my ARC (Advanced Reader Copy) **team**. As a member, you'll receive free copies of my upcoming **books** before they hit the shelves. Your honest **feedback** will be invaluable and help shape my work for future readers.

Becoming part of the **team** is an easy process:

• Click on "Join Review Team"

• Sign Up to BookSprout

• Get notified every time I release a new book

Check out the team at this link:

https://pxl.to/loganmindteam